D0943668

OPIATE ADDICTION:
ORIGINS AND TREATMENT

THE SERIES IN GENERAL PSYCHIATRY

Daniel X. Freedman · Consulting Editor

FISHER AND FREEDMAN · *Opiate Addiction: Origins and Treatment*

OPIATE ADDICTION:
ORIGINS AND TREATMENT

EDITED BY SEYMOUR FISHER

BOSTON UNIVERSITY SCHOOL OF MEDICINE

and ALFRED M. FREEDMAN

NEW YORK MEDICAL COLLEGE

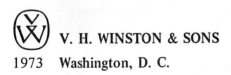 V. H. WINSTON & SONS

1973   Washington, D. C.

DISTRIBUTED BY THE HALSTED PRESS DIVISION OF

JOHN WILEY & SONS
New York   Toronto   London   Sydney

REF
RC 568
.06
063
Cop. 1

Copyright © 1974, by V. H. Winston & Sons, Inc.

All rights reserved. No part of this book may be reproduced by any form, by photostat, microform, retrieval system, or any other means, without the prior written permission of the publisher, except that reproduction in whole or in part is permitted for official use of the United States Government on the condition that the copyright notice is included with such official reproduction.

V. H. Winston & Sons, Inc., Publishers
1511 K St. N.W., Washington, D.C. 20005

Distributed solely by Halsted Press Division, John Wiley & Sons, Inc., New York.

ISBN 0-470-26153-6

Library of Congress Catalog Card Number: 73-19073

Printed in the United States of America

CONTENTS

NAT
R

PART II CLINICAL APPROACHES TO THE TREATMENT AND CONTROL OF OPIATE ADDICTION

LIST OF CONTRIBUTORS

Numbers in parentheses indicate the pages on which the authors' contributions begin.

John C. Ball, Addiction Sciences Center, Temple University, Philadelphia, Pennsylvania. (175)

Thomas H. Bewley, St. George's, St. Thomas', Tooting Bec Hospitals, London, England. (141)

Henry Brill, Pilgrim State Hospital, West Brentwood, New York. (171)

William E. Bunney, Jr., Division of Narcotic Addiction and Drug Abuse, National Institute of Mental Health, Rockville, Maryland. (43)

Joseph Cochin, Boston University School of Medicine, Boston, Massachusetts. (23)

Salvatore diMenza, Illinois Drug Abuse Program, University of Chicago, Chicago, Illinois. (185)

Matthew P. Dumont, Massachusetts Department of Mental Health, Boston, Massachusetts. (163)

Joel Elkes, Johns Hopkins University School of Medicine, Baltimore, Maryland. (123)

Max Fink, State University of New York-Stony Brook, Stony Brook, New York. (203)

Seymour Fisher, Boston University School of Medicine, Boston Massachusetts. (xi–Editor)

Alfred M. Freedman, New York Medical College, New York, New York. (xi, 225– Editor)

Daniel X. Freedman, University of Chicago, Chicago, Illinois. (3)

Harold Graff, Eastern Pennsylvania Psychiatric Institute, Philadelphia, Pennsylvania. (175)

Jerome H. Jaffe, Special Action Office for Drug Abuse Prevention,* Executive Office of the President, Washington, D.C. (127, 185)

Chris E. Johanson, University of Chicago, Chicago, Illinois. (77)

Herbert Kleber, Connecticut Mental Health Center, and Yale University School of Medicine, New Haven, Connecticut. (211)

Conan Kornetsky, Boston University School of Medicine, Boston, Massachusetts. (59)

David F. Musto, Yale University, New Haven, Connecticut. (93)

*Now Professor of Psychiatry at Columbia University.

Donald A. Overton,   Eastern Pennsylvania Psychiatric Institute, and Temple University Medical School, Philadelphia, Pennsylvania. (61)

Pierre F. Renault, University of Chicago, Chicago, Illinois. (185)

Charles R. Schuster, University of Chicago, Chicago, Illinois. (77)

Edward C. Senay, Illinois Drug Abuse Program, and University of Chicago, Chicago, Illinois. (185)

Stephen Szara, Center for Studies of Narcotic and Drug Abuse, National Institute of Mental Health, Rockville, Maryland. (43)

E. Leong Way, University of California School of Medicine, San Francisco, California. (99)

Abraham Wikler, University of Kentucky College of Medicine, Lexington, Kentucky. (7)

Joseph Zubin, New York State Department of Mental Hygiene, New York, New York. (223)

INTRODUCTION

This volume, based upon the December 1972 meeting of the American College of Neuropsychopharmacology, is particularly noteworthy. The all too prevalent conception of the College as being exclusively concerned with psychotropic drugs is negated. The College has never operated within such narrow confines and this volume indicates its broader scope.

Opiate addiction is a major problem in the United States, as well as elsewhere in the world. To comprehend its origin, to delineate its genesis, to develop rational methods of successful therapy, requires information from pharmacology, physiology, neurochemistry, sociology, law, psychology, and many other fields. In organizing the presentations published in this volume, the American College of Neuropsychopharmacology displayed the depth and breadth of its concerns and the varied interests of its membership.

In a troubled society, rhetoric may at times play an important role in focusing upon critical issues, but rhetoric alone cannot provide the solutions to those problems. Ultimately, these solutions can come only from a Solomonesque combination of clear, rational thought and empirical research findings.

The presentations comprising *Opiate Addiction: Origins and Treatment* make clear the complexity of the field and the necessity for major research endeavors. The possibilities of simple and ready solutions do not appear to be immediate. However, potentially productive and rewarding avenues are certainly available. This is of particular importance today, when there are frequent demands for instant results, with some even urging the virtual abandonment of all investigation and development in favor of hyperpunitive law-enforcement approaches. We hope this volume will stimulate and encourage further thought and research in this field.

The rapid publication of this volume was made possible by the efforts of two key people. We are grateful to Evelyn Stone for her indispensable editorial assistance, and we are especially indebted to Jody Harrison for her intelligence and tenacity in working with the editors and the contributors.

Seymour Fisher
Alfred M. Freedman

December, 1973

OPIATE ADDICTION:
ORIGINS AND TREATMENT

AMERICAN COLLEGE OF NEUROPSYCHOPHARMACOLOGY
OFFICERS—1972

President . . . .   ALFRED M. FREEDMAN, M.D.
President-elect . . . .   J. RICHARD WITTENBORN, Ph.D.
Vice President . . . .   FRIDOLIN SULSER, M.D.
Secretary-treasurer . . . .   DANIEL H. EFRON, M.D., Ph.D. (Deceased)
                                                    J. RICHARD WITTENBORN, Ph.D., pro tem
Assistant Secretary-treasurer . . . .   SOLOMON C. GOLDBERG, Ph.D.
Council . . . .   JOHN J. BURNS, Ph.D.
                                                    ARNOLD FRIEDHOFF, M.D.
                                                    LEO E. HOLLISTER, M.D.
                                                    SIDNEY MALITZ, M.D.
                                                    CHARLES SHAGASS, M.D.
Past President . . . .   JOSEPH ZUBIN, Ph.D.

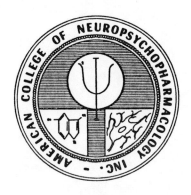

Program and Scientific Communications Committee

SEYMOUR FISHER, Ph.D., *Chairman*
KEITH F. KILLAM, Ph. D.
LOUIS LASAGNA, M.D.
ALLAN F. MIRSKY, Ph.D.
LARRY STEIN, Ph. D.

PART I PSYCHOSOCIAL AND PHARMACOLOGICAL ASPECTS OF OPIATE ADDICTION

SECTION 1
INTRODUCTION

Daniel X. Freedman
Department of Psychiatry, University of Chicago

Dr. Daniel Efron's indefatigable pursuit of excellence, his wish to wed pharmacology to psychopharmacology, knew the bounds of neither time, energy, ebullience nor enterprise. He completely gave himself to the job because he loved his mission and the scientific field and those in it. Both that love and the actual work of many laboratories and people, as well as the edited volumes, are a living epitaph to an enduringly good friend. It is appropriate that Abe Wikler—who assembled the first psychiatric text on psychoactive drugs, who helped to set the standards the scientific community must share, i.e., the value of inquiry over quick payoff and gimmickry—gives the first Daniel Efron Memorial Lecture.

Responsibility for coping with serious public health problems such as drug abuse can and should be broadly shared. Unfortunately, the profession and the addict have long had an uneasy and infrequent relationship. So, too, have enforcement agencies and medical practitioners. The authority to define legitimate medical practice with addicts has been at issue. Between 1921 and the present, law enforcement has exercised de facto primacy and prudent physicians have avoided prolonged treatment of the average addict who prototypically lived out of our sight, oscillating between the streets and jail. We must now begin to confront definitions which for the past 50 years have been so obscured.

In so doing, we should note that the physician who delivers services has a key obligation and role. Whatever the legalistic constraints, the reliable governance of the giving and getting of any drug is embedded in medical diagnosis and rests upon the integrity of the physician-patient relationship. With all its faults, the medical system is the one device by which the resources of scientific knowledge and judgment, consultation and evaluation can be brought to bear upon the individual case, and the risk and gain of pharmacotherapeutics balanced and monitored.

These issues are broader than "drug abuse" and accordingly will require our alertness and informed response. Drug use, misuse, and abuse occur with both licit and illicit drugs, in the context of medical practice as well as in recreational or group contexts. Underlying our society's striking preoccupation with the entire issue of drugs, whether or not they affect mood or mentation, there is enormous distrust and misunderstanding of the role of science and medicine.

As concern grows about improper use of products of technology and nature, scientists are charged with callousness and carelessness. While a legion of lay pharmacologists perform experiments never dared even by the midnight movie's mad scientist, useful medicines are tried not in the court of scientific debate but by exposé in the halls of Congress and in the scientific press (including *Time, Life, Playboy,* and the *New York Sunday Times*). The pill, cyclamates, mercurial tiffs about tuna, monosodium glutamate, stimulants for hyperkinetic children, as well as the current drugs of abuse, all keep the public pot boiling. There is sufficient evidence, then, of very real disarticulations in our capacity to think about and govern the giving, getting, and consumption of the products of nature and technology.

The role of the American College of Neuropsychopharmacology in assessing new knowledge may mean we cannot satisfy impossible—even Presidential—demands to eliminate evil, whether by molecular miracles, by computer-run systems tracking addicted little brothers, by such euphemisms for coercion as quarantine and mandatory medicating of populations at risk, or by fallible searches of urine (modern archaeology) to discover artifacts of yesterday's sins.

There are some paradoxical attitudes which render our society unable to design rational and trustworthy systems to govern these issues. Our egalitarian ethos permits the well-educated nonspecialist to expect instant explanations of complex issues which truly puzzle the involved research scientist. The schism of the "two cultures" which surround our attitudes on science and technology goes even deeper. In the formation of a "science policy," we encounter little general understanding of how scientific problems can be approached and solved, how inquiry is in fact mounted (rather than engineered), or how it is that the scientific conclusions of the moment may become abandoned launching pads in the search for the findings of the future. Neither the value, the limit, nor the intent of scientific method is often comprehended even by some technically facile as well as administratively prominent scientists. Among young and old, we encounter profound and dangerous beliefs that one's own experience is sufficient evidence to decide what is proper or good in the consuming of foods and drugs.

But the prevalent demand for instant knowledge or free access to any thought or experience is matched not only by demands for unscientific science, but by the requirement that government provide the consumer with absolute immunity from error when the products of technology are licitly marketed. Such paradoxical attitudes in turn probably do not enhance sensible or scientifically responsible decision-making by our harassed regulatory agencies.

While scientists are asked to produce knowledge—generally to back up one or another prejudice—we encounter a concerted attack on the systems by which authentic knowledge can be delivered. Budget-cutters, planners, and reformers, each beginning from a different premise, are busily in concert dismantling unversities and the stability of a system through which generations of teachers and students—through the processes of free inquiry—produce an occasional consequence of social value.

Experts protest, of course, that they should not be distrusted; yet they either remain aloof from teaching the public or—all too frequently—lend their fragmentary findings to various social movements and attempt to influence public behavior with premature publications. In the recent past, for example, we have seen that if a molecule produces pleasure, the Lord will punish the consumer with a dubious orthopedic disease known as "fractured chromosomes." Thus we must be rational in our approach to narcotics—a human needs problem tapping man's basic drives for pleasure and avoidance.

It appears, then, that we in the biomedical sciences face not only a crisis in the funding and delivery of health care, but also a crisis of trust, communication, and understanding. Underlying much of our disarray are a crisis in the delivery of authentic knowledge and a misunderstanding of the cumbersome apparatus necessary to it. It should be evident that the social aspects of pharmacology and biomedical science will require of all of us some attention, perspective, emphasis, and communication; it will be a burdensome but necessary tax on our time.

To clarify the contingent status of a scientific finding, the "wasted activity" bridging the gaps between occasional peaks of accomplishment, the unpredictability of the source of new knowledge, and the complexity with which ultimately simple operations are organized as sequences of behavior—these are tasks for public education. So, too, is maintenance of and respect for the system of inquirers ranging from the bench to the clinic, reciprocally posing problems and exchanging ideas—and adjudicating truth by critique and the logic of science. Some of these approaches must be applied to drug abuse.

The question whether a drug issue is basically a legal, economic, or health problem is a complex one. Essentially, a society must regulate its drugs by establishing customs, controlling both the manufacture of and the access to drugs, or attempting to control the behavior of persons. But it is striking that we have never looked at our total drug network in a systematic way, nor have we assembled under any responsible auspices the gamut of involved persons (from manufacturers to educators and scientists, and from distributors to consumers) to assess our needs and the consequences of randomly proposed solutions.

These defects in our total societal capacity to regulate medicines tend to make us highly vulnerable, eliciting a shortsighted response to the concerns about currently unpopular drugs and persons using them. The piecemeal approach to drug abuse simply makes such fissures in our body politic more visible. Within the biomedical sciences we should recall that, while the rules of evidence belong to science, what is and is not legitimate research and medical practice is ultimately defined by society. The role of inquiry plays a part in this process, and its integrity and vitality rests on its freedom, its intrinsic limitations, as well as responsiveness to general social concerns. This, then, is the overall task and significance of our deliberations.

DYNAMICS OF DRUG DEPENDENCE: IMPLICATIONS OF A CONDITIONING THEORY FOR RESEARCH AND TREATMENT[1]

Abraham Wikler
University of Kentucky School of Medicine

INTRODUCTION

In successive formulations of the definition of "drug dependence," the World Health Organization (WHO) has stressed, to an increasing degree, a feature common to all types of drug dependence, namely:

> ... a particular state of mind that is termed *psychic dependence*. In this situation, there is a feeling of satisfaction and a psychic drive that require periodic or continuous administration of the drug to produce pleasure or avoid discomfort. Indeed, this mental state is the most powerful of all the factors involved in chronic intoxication with psychotropic drugs, and with certain types of drugs it may be the only factor involved, even in the most intense craving and perpetuation of compulsive abuse. . . . Physical dependence is a powerful factor in reinforcing the influence of psychic dependence upon continuing drug use or relapse to drug use after attempted withdrawal [4].

Defined in this manner, the concept of psychic dependence has a strong common-sense appeal, since it is consonant with the pain-pleasure principle—a principle which, since time immemorial, has been taken for granted as a sufficient explanation of behavior by the man in the street, "idealist" philosophers, and introspectively inclined psychiatrists and psychologists. The pain-pleasure principle, however, is empty tautology, for its perfect circularity becomes apparent after a moment's reflection. Nor can one infer, from the cited definition alone, just what the tangible variables are, of which "psychic" (as opposed to "physical") and "dependence" are functions. However, analysis of a more detailed description of psychic dependence [3] suggests that this term

[1] Supported, in part, by NIMH grants MH 13194 and MH 17748.

refers to reinforcement of drug-using behavior consequent on interactions between certain pharmacological (i.e., physical) actions of a drug and certain organismic variables that had *not* been engendered by previous doses of that drug, and to reinforcement of drug-using behavior consequent on social reinforcement, in which a "need to belong," rather than the pharmacological actions of the drug, plays the dominant role. In contrast, physical dependence clearly refers to reinforcement of drug-using behavior consequent on interactions between certain pharmacological actions of a drug and organismic variables that *had been* engendered by previous doses of the drug. A further implication is that for each kind of interaction there is a corresponding subjective state which "drives" the user to renewed self-administration of the drug. Thus, in a psychically dependent person, each self-administered dose of the drug is said to alter—in a "pleasurable" direction, of course—an "unpleasant mood" state that was the consequence, not of the effects of previous doses of the drug, but of *antecedent* "anxiety," "depression," "boredom," and the like. At the same time, such drug use (together with affirmation of popular beliefs about drug-produced "highs," "thrills," "rushes," etc.) gains for the user acceptance into a dominant or "deviant" social group that provides him with many other kinds of reinforcements. In the tolerant and physically dependent user, however, each dose of the drug is said merely to stave off or suppress the "pain and suffering" associated with abstinence phenomena. Finally, the WHO definitions imply that relapse, even long after drug withdrawal, is due to "craving," aroused by the memory of the "pleasures" experienced formerly in the state of psychic dependence; presumably, the "pain and suffering" associated previously with physical dependence is somehow forgotten, even though the literature is replete with accounts of the "agonies of the damned" reported retrospectively by former drug users themselves.

CONDITIONING FACTORS IN OPIOID DEPENDENCE

In an attempt to devise an operationally definable conceptual framework for research which would provide "cells" for all the known and putative variables of which drug dependence may be a function, I have elected to use a conditioning theory of opioid dependence as a model [36, 37, 42]. Drug dependence is defined as "habitual, nonmedically indicated drug-seeking and drug-using behaviour which is contingent for its maintenance upon pharmacological and usually, but not necessarily, upon social reinforcement [40]." So defined, the strength of drug dependence may be measured by its resistance to extinction or suppression. Pharmacological reinforcement is viewed as the resultant of interactions between certain pharmacological effects of the drug and "sources of reinforcement"—i.e., organismic variables upon the existence of which the reinforcing properties of the drug are contingent. Pharmacological reinforcement is said to be "direct" if such sources of reinforcement had not been engendered by the drug itself, or "indirect" if the contrary is true. Furthermore, sources of direct pharmacological reinforcement may be "intrinsic" (built into the central nervous system) or "developmental" (acquired in the course of personality development or otherwise). In our present state of knowledge, the only example of a source of indirect pharmacological reinforcement is the changes in the central nervous system that are adduced to explain physical dependence [41]. But the concept is meant to include other, yet-to-be-discovered kinds of drug-engendered organismic variables, interaction of which with the drug may be found to be reinforcing. Also, pharmacological reinforcement, direct or indirect, may be "primary" (unconditioned) or "secondary" (conditioned).

THEORY OF RELAPSE

Details of this conceptual scheme are presented in Table 1. Space does not permit discussion of all the cells in the Table, but it should be noted that "craving" (indicated here by the equivalent phrase, "need a fix") and relapse long after "detoxification" are attributed to reactivation, by previously conditioned extero- and/or interoceptive stimuli, of classically conditioned central "counteradaptations" to the original, agonistic effects of opioids, and of any neural processes that may underlie operant conditioning of drug-seeking behavior.

That morphine-abstinence phenomena *can* be conditioned in animals has been demonstrated by two methods: (a) pairing a specific environment with the relatively slow onset and progression to peak intensity of the abstinence syndrome that follows abrupt withdrawal of morphine—the method used in our laboratory [38, 49]; and (b) pairing a discrete stimulus with the nalorphine-precipitated morphine-abstinence syndrome—the method used by Goldberg and Schuster [6, 7]. I might add that some evidence of the conditionability of the nalorphine-precipitated abstinence syndrome in man [45] was obtained some 20 years ago in our original studies on the precipitation of abstinence syndromes by nalorphine in experimental subjects receiving multiple daily doses of morphine, methadone, or heroin [47]. In five such subjects, partially tolerant to morphine or methadone administered subcutaneously on a fixed 4-times-daily schedule by ward aides, single doses of nalorphine, given on an irregular schedule by my technician, always provoked typical opioid-abstinence phenomena within 2-3 minutes after subcutaneous injection. Later in the course of the study, saline trials occasionally substituted for nalorphine but also given by my technician evoked, during the first 2-3 weeks of such trials, complaints of "hot and cold all over," cramps, nausea and/or gagging, and frequently objective responses, including yawning, lacrimation, rhinorrhea, and mydriasis, within 30 minutes after subcutaneous injection. Then such responses to saline rapidly declined: by personal inquiry I found that the subjects, all of them highly experienced "hustlers," had been watching each other, and had come to the (correct) conclusion that if the first one to receive my technician's injection on a given

TABLE 1
Opioid Dependence Reinforcement Processes

Reinforcing processes	Sources	Reinforcing events	Behavior
I. SOCIAL Street-corner society; slum "big shots"; cultist rituals & beliefs	Need to belong; boredom; anhedonia; anomie; hostility to "establishment"	Acceptance by deviant sub-culture	Drug-taking in accordance with rituals; affirmation of cultist beliefs
II. PRIMARY PHARMACOLOGICAL A. Direct (nondrug-engendered = psychic dependence)	1. Intrinsic (cerebral drug-sensitive "reward" systems?) 2. Developmental (personality): anxiety in *particular* situations	1. Relatively nonspecific drug effects (release or blockade of NE, DA, ACh, etc. in brain) 2. *Specific* pattern of agonistic actions of opioid drugs	1. Subjective: "high"; "thrills" (i.v. only) Objective: elated behavior 2. Subjective: "content"; "relaxed", "coasting" Objective: nodding; leveling of performance
B. Indirect (drug-engendered = physical dependence)	Early abstinence changes (manifest or detectable by subject's cerebral sensors); restlessness, etc.	Suppression of early abstinence by next dose of opioid NOTE: Tolerance has developed to "directly" reinforcing effects of opioids	Subjective: craving and satisfaction of craving Objective: "hustling" for opioids; increasing dose and frequency of opioid-taking (*appetitively* conditioned behavior)

III. SECONDARY PHARMACOLOGICAL			
A. Direct	Classically conditioned CNS changes (counter-adaptive to agonistic effects of opioids)	Agonistic effects of opioids as in II A & B. However, after II A *and* B, suppression of conditioned abstinence is more reinforcing.	Subjective: A. "Feel blue"; "disgusted." B. "Feel sick"; "got the flu"; "need a fix."
B. Indirect (both A & B, "exteroceptive" and "interoceptive")	A. Conditioned inhibition of CNS "reward" systems		Objective: A. Depressive behavior. B. Signs of opioid abstinence (conditioned); renewed "hustling" RELAPSE
	B. Conditioned abstinence changes		

"Reinforcement" = interaction between sources of reinforcement and reinforcing events. Note.–Reprinted, with permission, from A. Wikler: Sources of reinforcement for drug using behavior–A theoretical formulation. Pharmacology and the Future of Man. Proceedings of the 5th International Congress on Pharmacology, San Francisco 1972. Volume 1 in press (Basel: Karger, 1973).

day did not get "sick" within 2-3 minutes, the "shot" for that day was a "blank." At the time, I castigated myself for not having employed a more sophisticated experimental design. In retrospect, however, the observation that decoding of the experimental design by these subjects altered the properties of the conditioned stimulus attests to the power of cognitive labeling in man, and suggests that verbal psychotherapy, if properly employed, might be useful in facilitating extinction of conditioned abstinence, in conjunction with behavioral extinction procedures (see below).

Returning to the animal data, a most important point is that in rats the conditioned abstinence sign we studied, namely, increased frequency of "wet dog" shakes in the conditioned environment, persisted for 155 days (5 months) after withdrawal of morphine, and in the monkeys studied by Goldberg and Schuster the conditioned nalorphine-precipitated abstinence phenomena, namely, transitory suppression of lever-pressing for food, vomiting, salivation, and bradycardia, could be elicited for up to 120 days after withdrawal of morphine.

Operant conditioning of drug self-administration in animals has been demonstrated by many investigators, and it has been shown with both the drinking and self-injection techniques that such operantly trained animals will relapse [14, 24, 32, 35]. However, these studies do not settle the question whether such relapse is related to previous indirect pharmacological reinforcement ("physical dependence") or to previous direct pharmacological reinforcement (one of the meanings of "psychic dependence"), of which an example cited in the literature is the self-maintenance on very small intravenous doses of morphine by naive monkeys [52]. However, Jones and Prada [10] found that, while most dogs will not initiate self-injection of morphine, such animals will maintain their addiction by self-injection after they have been made physically dependent by passive injections of morphine, and will relapse promptly after morphine withdrawal and removal from the operant chamber for as long as 6 months. All we can say at present is that previous physical dependence can be a powerful factor in facilitating relapse. Whether such facilitation is due to protracted abstinence [8, 19, 20], to conditioning processes, or to a combination of both, is a problem for future investigation. In our own studies, rats with previous physical dependence relapsed in choice drinking tests (etonitazene [48] solution vs. water) at intervals of 1-3 weeks over a period of about 1 year after withdrawal of morphine, even without "formal" operant conditioning [50]. However, the persistent potency (for at least 137 days after morphine withdrawal) of a secondary (conditioned) "exteroceptive" reinforcer generated by previous temporal contiguity between such a stimulus and suppression of early morphine-abstinence phenomena suggests the possibility that, even without observer-manipulated operant training, opioid-seeking behavior can become "interoceptively" conditioned in subjects who undergo the continuous cycle of early opioid abstinence and its suppression by the next dose of the drug [51].

IMPLICATIONS FOR RESEARCH AND TREATMENT

I have already alluded to two problems that require further investigation: the roles of protracted abstinence and of conditioning factors in the genesis of relapse. The latter, however, is part of a more general problem—namely, that of conditioning of drug effects, both classical and operant. Emboldened by the data and ideas of Konorski [12], Miller and DiCara [22], and Miller [21]. I venture to propose [43], at least to simplify the problem of drug conditioning, that the neural mechanisms of classical and operant conditioning are the same, the phenomenological differences being due to the differences in what is "reinforced": a "reflexly" elicited unconditioned response (UR) in the case of classical conditioning or an "emitted" UR in the case of operant conditioning. The *reinforcing event* in *both* cases is the delayed activation of "rewarding" or "punishing" limbic structures that follows presentation of the unconditioned stimulus (US—in operant terms, the "reinforcer") and the UR which the US elicits. If this assumption is correct, then two behaviors are conditioned in operant conditioning: the emitted behavior in which the experimenter is interested, and the UR elicited by the reinforcer (US) in which he is not interested (although Shapiro [30], for example, recorded not only lever-presses but also parotid salivary secretion during acquisition of food-reinforced responding by dogs). Stein [29] has offered an interesting suggestion on how delayed activation of limbic structures may be the critical reinforcing event:

Pairing an operant response with reward may be viewed as an instance of Pavlovian conditioning. Response-related stimuli (environmental as well as internal) are the conditioned stimulus and reward is the unconditioned stimulus. By virtue of the pairing, the medial forebrain "go" mechanism is conditioned to response-related stimuli. Thus, on future occasions, any tendency to engage in the previously rewarded behaviour initiates facilitatory feedback by activation of the "go" mechanism, and thereby increases the probability that the response will run off to completion. In the case of punishment, periventricular activity is conditioned to stimuli associated with the punished operant. This decreases the probability that the operant will be emitted in the future because feedback from the "stop" mechanism will tend to inhibit the behaviour.

In the special case of those behaviors we call "drug effects," I have proposed [43] that what becomes conditioned are central "processing" events consequent to the initial (agonistic) effects of drugs at neuronal receptor sites in the afferent arms of "reflex" circuits, broadly conceived to include not only the familiar bulbospinal reflexes, but also complex afferent-processing-efferent and feedback networks, the afferent neurons of which may lie outside the pia mater (exteroceptors and interoceptors such as baroreceptors and chemoreceptors) or at various loci in the brain (chemoreceptors, osmoreceptors, thermoreceptors). In this view, certain drug effects *are* "reflex" or "adaptive" responses to their initial effects at afferent receptor sites (e.g., morphine emesis [33, 34]), while other drug effects represent compensatory (feedback) responses to initial effects of such drugs at peripheral effector sites [17]. In these cases, pairing a "neutral" conditional stimulus (CS) with administration of the drug on repeated occasions results in conditioned responses CRs that mimic the URs [27, 11, 17]. In other cases, such as those of drugs acting on post-synaptic receptors in autonomic ganglia, compensatory, centrally processed responses are *developed* after repeated pairings of the CS and US, and the CRs that emerge are *opposite* in direction to the URs. For example, repeated pairing of a CS with subcutaneous injection of atropine (in dogs and cats) eventually results in profuse salivation on presentation of the CS, which can be blocked by atropine, Ditran, or propranolol [13, 16, 36]. It is still not clear whether this "paradoxical" CR represents unconditioned potentiation (by supersensitization of the chronically atropinized salivary glands to acetylcholine and catecholamines [5]) of a specific conditioned, central adaptation to peripheral blockade of salivary secretion, or a nonspecific conditioned, central adaptive response to "noxious" stimulation. But in either case the phenomenon illustrates the principle that with drugs acting at effector sites it is an unconditionally acquired adaptive response that becomes conditioned. Conditioning of unconditionally acquired adaptive responses is also illustrated by the conditioning of hypoglycemic responses—to saccharine in man—reported by Kun and Horvath [15] and by the remarkable experiments of Roffman and Lal [28]. The latter found that in mice, after repeated pairing of a CS with reduced oxygen tension which unconditionally produced hypothermia and prolongation of hexobarbital narcosis, presentation of the CS alone evoked hyperthermia and shortening of hexobarbital narcosis. Apparently, however, not all unconditionally acquired feedback circuits are "adaptive," at least from a teleological perspective. Thus, in the rat, Woods and his coworkers [54] were able to condition the hypoglycemic effects of subcutaneously injected insulin and found evidence of insulin-like activity in the blood just before the appearance of conditioned hypoglycemia. Also, Woods et al. [53] reported that, after repeated subcutaneous injections of tolbutamide, injection of the tolbutamide vehicle alone evoked conditioned insulin secretion and hypoglycemia. Interestingly, they mention that, "Since conditioned hypoglycemia has been found to require intact vagus nerves and to be eliminated with atropine . . . , the implication is that the animals can be made to neurally increase their insulin output." In any case, adaptive or not, these data likewise indicate that in the cases of the USs, insulin and tolbutamide, what becomes conditioned is not, respectively, the transport of glucose across membranes of glucose-utilizing cells or the direct stimulation of pancreatic islet beta cells, but a central processing event mediated to the pancreatic islets by the vagus nerve; this results in secretion of more insulin, and hence in conditioned hypoglycemia—for what "purpose," we cannot yet say.

Applying these concepts to the problem of drug dependence, we can postulate further: as drug administrations are continued in frequent temporal contiguity with certain exteroceptive and/or interoceptive stimuli, these CSs come to elicit, as CRs, *successive* unconditioned adaptations and counteradaptations to the initial (agonistic) actions of the drug at receptor sites in afferent arms of neural reflex (broad sense) circuits [43]. In this view, the CRs that develop in the allegedly non-tolerant and non-physically dependent "joy popper" can be expected to be different from those that develop in the tolerant and physically dependent "addict." But in both cases the consequence of this view is that the CRs are opposite in direction to the initial reflex responses to the agonistic effects of the drug, and are experienced as "dysphoria" (Table 1). Inasmuch as in self-injectors such behavior had also become operantly conditioned, evocation of such classically conditioned counteradaptive responses by the CSs, even long after detoxification, can be expected to result in relapse.

Another consequence of this view is that the sharp distinction usually made between psychic dependence (direct pharmacological reinforcement) and physical dependence (indirect pharmacological reinforcement) becomes untenable. Thus, it may be questioned whether, after the first few doses of any of the drugs of abuse, including those said not to produce physical dependence (amphetamines, cocaine, cannabis products), the drug-reinforcing processes remain "direct" (i.e., nondrug-engendered). In the case of morphine, it has been demonstrated that in naive chronic spinal dogs, hindlimb abstinence phenomena can be precipitated by nalorphine given 1 hour after a single dose of morphine [46]. In man, clear-cut abstinence phenomena can be evoked by nalorphine (15 mg) after administration of morphine (15 mg), methadone (10 mg), or heroin (15 mg) 4 times daily for as little as 2 or 3 days [47]. The interactions between opioids and neurotransmitters are still obscure, but it is known that many psychoactive drugs release, block reuptake of, or otherwise alter the effects of neurotransmitters at their receptor sites, and that the central nervous system is equipped with elaborate neural, positive and negative feedback circuits [1] which serve to counteract such direct drug effects. Perhaps such neural feedback circuits tend to "overshoot," and thereby generate new sources of reinforcement, with or without those abstinence signs we have learned to recognize (e.g., the abstinence syndromes that follow abrupt withdrawal of opioids, barbiturates, or ethanol after chronic intoxication with these drugs). Certainly, in the case of amphetamine—long considered a drug that does not produce physical dependence—the prolonged "rebound" REM sleep that ensues after its abrupt withdrawal [25, 26], as well as the succeeding transitory bulimia followed by affective depression, *are* abstinence phenomena, which were not recognized as such for so long because the patient, being asleep, did not complain. In terms of the pain-pleasure principle, is the "speed freak" impelled to self-inject amphetamine in closely spaced doses, and to relapse in the Haight-Ashbury environment after "crashing" there, because of the memories of the "highs" produced by the first dose or of the "lows" that followed? Similar questions may be asked about cocaine self-administration and marijuana smoking. However, answers to these questions in terms of the pain-pleasure principle will not be meaningful; rather, the answers should be sought in terms of the biochemical-neurophysiological mechanisms that are involved in the development of successive counteradaptations to the initial receptor-actions of such drugs, and in reinforcement.

Some implications of this conditioning theory for treatment of drug-dependent persons in general [39] and of opioid-dependent persons in particular [44] have been discussed *in extenso* elsewhere. Suffice it here to point out that mere detoxification, with or without conventional psychotherapy and prolonged retention in a drug-free environment, does not result in extinction of the conditioned responses, any more than satiating a rat with food (i.e., reducing its hunger drive) and keeping it away from the operant cage for a period of time will "cure" it of its lever-pressing habit, which it had acquired previously under conditions of food deprivation [38]. Rather, what is needed in post-detoxification treatment is repeated elicitation of the conditioned responses by appropriate conditioned stimuli and *active* extinction of them by programmed self-injection of the drug of dependence under conditions that preclude its reinforcing effects. Verbal psychotherapy might be utilized effectively to hasten extinction (*vide supra*) if it is directed toward "cognitive relabeling" of the conditioned responses, instead of toward resolution of alleged oral fixations and the like. In the particular case of detoxified opioid-dependent persons, a promising means of achieving extinction is afforded by the availability of long-lasting, orally effective narcotic antagonists [18], which not only prevent opioid "euphoria," but are even more important in preventing suppression of opioid abstinence phenomena by opioids and the renewed development of physical dependence even after repeated doses of opioids—i.e., they prevent reinforcement of conditioned abstinence and of conditioned opioid-seeking behavior.

In the practical application of these principles, the detoxified and narcotic-antagonist-maintained patient, *while still in the hospital*, should be exposed to laboratory facsimiles of his "bad associates," and to anxiety-producing situations which, mimicking the stimuli to which he had been exposed while "hustling" for opioids previously, are likely to evoke conditioned abstinence. The patient should be required to self-inject genuine, guaranteed "pure" heroin repeatedly with all the rituals to which he had been accustomed, in doses which are greater than those he would be likely to obtain on the street, but which are insufficient to overcome the narcotic-antagonist blockade. It can be expected that, eventually, the patient will refuse to self-inject heroin further, and the laboratory facsimiles of his presumed exteroceptive and interoceptive conditioned stimuli will cease to evoke signs of conditioned abstinence. Then, the patient may be discharged from the hospital, but he should continue to be maintained on the antagonist in his home environment, with its "real-life" conditioned stimuli (including secondary reinforcers). Very likely, responding to these conditioned stimuli, the patient will resort to self-injection of "bags" of heroin, but it can be expected that such spontaneous recovery from extinction will be short-lived, because of previous active extinction in the hospital and continued narcotic-antagonist blockade. A priori, it is difficult to estimate how long narcotic-antagonist blockade should be maintained, but inasmuch as protracted abstinence can last for approximately 10 months after abrupt withdrawal of morphine following experimental chronic morphine intoxication in man [19], 1 year would seem reasonable, provided that randomly taken urine samples remain drug-free during the last few months.

Equally important is the problem of retraining the detoxified patient to "hustle" for socially approved reinforcers in the drug-free "internal state," after having successfully deprived him of both the reinforcers (primary and secondary) and the opioid internal state generated during years of opioid dependence. In this connection, a fact that was recently confirmed [23] should be more seriously considered—namely, that the vast majority of opioid post-addicts are people with various forms of psychopathology, the most common being "psychopathy" or, more politely, "sociopathy." One characteristic of psychopaths is their inability to delay gratification (i.e., to emit sustained, goal-directed activity under conditions of delayed reinforcement and consummation). Theoretically, an ideal vocation for such a person would be one that "paid off" immediately on successful completion of a task, but it is difficult to think of such occupations in our society, other than illegal or shady ones. Perhaps behavior-modification therapies could be devised for training psychopaths to work for reinforcements delivered at progressively longer fixed intervals and to delay their consumption for progressively longer periods. Also, we should note the possibility that, as in the rat [2, 7a], some socially useful behaviors that the patient had acquired in the opioid internal state are rapidly extinguished in the drug-free internal state. Should research demonstrate that state-dependent learning ("dissociated learning") applies to the opioid-dependent state in man, then such socially useful behaviors may have to be relearned, through appropriate therapy.

PREVENTION OF DRUG DEPENDENCE

From all the foregoing it is apparent that, in very large measure, drug dependence is a consequence of certain rather subtle pharmacological actions of "drugs of abuse," coupled with equally subtle conditioning processes. Therefore, control of drug availability, to the extent that this is possible practically, must be a *sine qua non* for prevention of drug dependence. However, the historical association between the development of drug mythologies, from the allegedly nonaddicting properties of heroin [31] and, later, meperidine [9] to the contemporary "psychedelic" preoccupations of so many of our youth and their older apologists, and the spread of drug abuse and drug dependence in the United States suggests, if it does not prove, that social reinforcement plays a significant role in bringing the host and the agent together. Dealing with this factor in the etiology of drug dependence takes us beyond the confines of scientific discourse, into the area of value judgments: Do we envisage with equanimity a society, say in 1984, whose members find their major primary reinforcers in psychotropic drugs and their secondary reinforcers in drug-cult beliefs and practices [39]? If not, then, as psychopharmacologists, we should do what we can to dispel the magical thinking about drug effects that permeates our society. At the very least, we can refrain from falling in line with the popular argot which refers to drug effects in such seductive but meretricious terms as "highs" or "psychedelic experiences." We can also be honest enough to say that drugs which alter the mind do so by altering the brain—a difference that should make a difference to any thoughtful person—and that even drugs which do not produce gross evidence of organic brain damage (like heroin or marihuana) can, nevertheless, produce serious behavioral damage after long-term use. To be sure, social reinforcement of drug use is a function not only of mythologies about drug effects, but also of cultural, political, and economic conditions. In these areas, however, our roles as psychopharmacologists do not particularly qualify us to express other than personal value judgments.

SUMMARY

Self-administration of psychoactive drugs is often initiated through social reinforcement (by peer groups, folkloristic and literary mystiques about drug effects, and/or iatrogenically). After the first or first few doses, successive central counteradaptive changes (CCCs) develop unconditionally in response to the initial (receptor-site) actions of the drug and their "reflex" consequences (signs of drug effects), thereby generating a homeostatic "need." Temporary reduction of this need by each successive self-administration of the drug in temporal contiguity with frequently recurring extero- and interoceptive stimuli (CSs) results in increasing probability of occurrence (reinforcement) both of the CCCs and of drug self-administering behavior in the presence of the CSs (appetitive conditioning). Continued drug use results in progressive multiplication and intensification of CCCs (manifested as "abstinence syndromes" if the drugs are withheld), as well as of the reinforcement and conditioning processes. Detoxification (DTX) alone does not result in extinction (EXT) of conditioned responses so generated, and subsequent relapse may be due to evocation by such CSs of "conditioned abstinence" (CA) and conditioned drug-seeking behavior. In the treatment of opioid post-addicts, EXT should be initiated while the patient is still in hospital by repeated elicitation of CA by "simulated" CSs, coupled with programmed opioid self-injection under narcotic-antagonist blockade, and continued until the patient desists. After discharge, and with continued maintenance on the antagonist (for about a year), exposure to "real-life" CSs and self-injection of illicit opioids may result in completion of EXT. Concomitantly, socially acceptable reinforcers should be generated by behavioral therapy and psychotherapy, cognizant of psychopathologies prevalent among post-addicts and theoretically possible consequences of "state-dependent learning." Prevention of drug dependence requires control of availability of psychotropic drugs and debunking of drug-culture mythologies, including the meretricious language in which these are expressed ("highs," "turning on," "psychedelic experiences," etc.).

REFERENCES

1. Axelrod, J. Neural and hormonal control of catecholamine synthesis. In I. J. Kopin (Ed.), *Neurotransmitters. Research Publications.* Ass. Nerv. Ment. Dis., Vol. 50. Baltimore: Williams & Wilkins, 1972.
2. Belleville, R. E. Control of behavior by drug-produced internal stimuli. *Psychopharmacologia* (Berl.), **5**, 95–105, 1964.
3. Cameron, D. C. Abuse of alcohol and drugs: concepts and planning. *Wld. Hlth. Org. Chronicle*, **25**, 8–16, 1971.
4. Eddy, N. B., Halbach, H., Isbell, H., & Seevers, M. H. Drug dependence: its significance and characteristics. In P. H. Blachly (Ed.), *Drug abuse. Data and debate* (Appendix A). Springfield: Thomas, 1970.
5. Emmelin, N. Supersensitivity following "pharmacological denervation." *Pharmacol. Rev.*, **13**, 17–37, 1961.
6. Goldberg, S. R., & Schuster, C. R. Conditioned suppression by a stimulus associated with nalorphine in morphine-dependent monkeys. *J. Exper. Anal. Behav.*, **10**, 235–242, 1967.
7. Goldberg, S. R., & Schuster, C. R. Conditioned nalorphine-induced abstinence changes: persistence in post-dependent monkeys. *J. Exper. Anal. Behav.*, **14**, 33–46, 1970.
7a. Hill, H. E., Jones B. E., & Bell, E. C. State dependent control of discrimination by morphine and pentobarbital. *Psychopharmacologia* (Berl.), **22**, 305–313, 1971.
8. Himmelsbach, C. K. Clinical studies of drug addiction: physical dependence, withdrawal and recovery. *Arch. Int. Med.*, **69**, 766–772, 1942.
9. Isbell, H., & White, W. M. Clinical characteristics of addiction. *Amer. J. Med.*, **14**, 558–565, 1953.
10. Jones, B. E., & Prada, J. A. Relapse to morphine (CRC) use in dog. *Fed. Proc.*, **31**, 551 Abs., 1972.
11. Kleitman, N., & Crisler, G. A quantitative study of a salivary conditioned reflex. *Amer. J. Physiol.*, **79**, 571–614, 1927.
12. Konorski, J. *Integrative activity of the brain. An interdisciplinary approach.* Chicago: University of Chicago Press, 1967.
13. Korol, B., Sletten, I. W., & Brown, M. L. Conditioned physiological adaptation to anticholinergic drugs. *Amer. J. Physiol.*, **211**, 911–914, 1966.
14. Kumar, R., & Stolerman, I. P. Resumption of morphine self-administration by ex-addict rats: an attempt to modify tendencies to relapse. *J. Comp. Physiol. Psychol.*, **78**, 457–465, 1972.
15. Kun, E., & Horvath, I. The influence of oral saccharin on blood sugar. *Proc. Soc. Exp. Biol.* (N.Y.), **66**, 175–177, 1947.
16. Lang, W. J., Brown, M. L., Gershon, S., & Korol, B. Classical and physiologic adaptive conditioned responses to anticholinergic drugs in conscious dogs. *Int. J. Neuropharmacol.*, **6**, 311–315, 1966.
17. Lang, W. J., Ross, P., & Glover, A. Conditional responses induced by hypotensive drugs. *Europ. J. Pharmacol.*, **2**, 169–174, 1967.
18. Martin, W. R., Gorodetzky, C. W., & McClane, T. K. An experimental study in the treatment of narcotic addicts with cyclazocine. *Clin. Pharmacol. Ther.*, **7**, 455–465, 1966.

19. Martin, W. R., & Jasinski, D. R. Physiological parameters of morphine dependence in man–tolerance, early abstinence, protracted abstinence. *J. Psychiat. Res.*, 7, 9–17, 1969.

20. Martin, W. R., Wikler, A., Eades, C. G., & Pescor, F. T. Tolerance to and physical dependence on morphine in the rat. *Psychopharmacologia* (Berl.), 4, 247–260, 1963.

21. Miller, N. E. Learning of visceral and glandular responses. *Science*, 163, 434–444, 1969.

22. Miller, N. E., & DiCara, L. V. Instrumental learning of urine formation by rats; changes in renal blood flow. *Amer. J. Physiol.*, 215, 677–683, 1968.

23. Monroe, J. J., Ross, W. F., & Berzins, J. I. The decline of the addict as "psychopath": implications for community care. *Int. J. Addictions*, 6, 601–608, 1971.

24. Nichols, J. R., Headlee, C. P., & Coppock, H. W. Drug addiction. I. Addiction by escape training. *J. Amer. Pharmaceut. Ass.* (sci. ed.), 45, 788–791, 1956.

25. Oswald, I. Effects on sleep of amphetamine and its derivatives. In E. Costa & S. Garattini (Eds.), *International symposium on amphetamine and related compounds*. New York: Raven Press, 1970.

26. Oswald, I., & Thacore, V. R. Amphetamine and phenmetrazine addiction. Physical abnormalities in the abstinence syndrome. *Brit. Med. J.*, 2, 427–431, 1963.

27. Pavlov, I. P. *Conditioned reflexes. An investigation of the physiological activity of the cerebral cortex*. Trans. & ed. by G. V. Anrep. London: Oxford University Press, 1927. (New York: Dover, 1960.)

28. Roffman, M., & Lal, H. Voluntary control of hepatic drug metabolism: a case of behavioral drug tolerance. Volunteer Abstracts, 5th International Congress on Pharmacology, San Francisco, July 1972. (Abstract #1167)

29. Stein, L. Amphetamine and neural reward mechanisms. In H. Steinberg, A. V. S. de Reuck, & J. Knight (Eds.), *Ciba foundation symposium on animal behaviour and drug action*. London: J. & A. Churchill, 1964.

30. Shapiro, M. M. Respondent salivary conditioning during operant lever pressing in dogs. *Science*, 132, 619–620, 1960.

31. Taylor, W. J. R., Chambers, C. D., & Bowling, C. E. Addiction and the community (narcotic substitution therapy). *Int. J. Pharmacol.*, 6, 28–39, 1972.

32. Thompson, T., & Ostlund, W. Susceptibility to re-addiction as a function of the addiction and withdrawal environment. *J. Comp. Physiol. Psychol.*, 59, 388–392, 1965.

33. Wang, S. C., & Borison, H. L. The vomiting center. A critical experimental analysis. *Arch. Neurol. Psychiat.* (Chicago), 63, 928–941, 1950.

34. Wang, S. C., & Glaviano, V. V. Locus of emetic action of morphine and hydergine in dogs. *J. Pharmacol. Exp. Ther.*, 111, 329–334, 1954.

35. Weeks, J. R., & Collins, R. J. Patterns of intravenous self-injection by morphine-addicted rats. In A. Wikler (Ed.), *The addictive states. Research Publications.* Ass. Nerv. Ment. Dis., Vol. 46. Baltimore: Williams & Wilkins, 1968.

36. Wikler, A. Recent progress in research on the neurophysiological basis of morphine addiction. *Amer. J. Psychiat.*, 105, 329–338, 1948.

37. Wikler, A. On the nature of addiction and habituation. *Brit. J. Addiction*, 57, 73–80, 1961.

38. Wikler, A. Conditioning factors in opiate addiction and relapse. In D. I. Wilner & G. G. Kassebaum (Eds.), *Narcotics*. New York: McGraw-Hill, 1965.

39. Wikler, A. Some implications of conditioning theory for problems of drug abuse. In P. Blachy (Ed.), *Drug abuse. Data and debate*. Springfield: Thomas, 1970. (Reprinted with permission in *Behav. Sci.*, 16, 92–97, 1971.)

40. Wikler, A. Present status of the concept of drug dependence. *Psychol. Med.* (London), 1, 377–380, 1971.

41. Wikler, A. Theories related to physical dependence. In S. J. Mulé & H. Brill (Eds.), *The chemical and biological aspects of drug dependence*. Cleveland: Chemical Rubber Co. Press, 1972.
42. Wikler, A. Sources of reinforcement for drug using behavior. A theoretical formulation. Abstracts (Invited Papers, pp. 135-136), 5th International Congress on Pharmacology, San Francisco, 23-28, July 1972. In *Proceedings of the Fifth International Congress on Pharmacology*. Basel: Karger, in press.
43. Wikler, A. Conditioning of successive adaptive responses to the initial effects of drugs. Presented in the Symposium on Psychophysiological Aspects of Drug Addiction, Society for Psychophysiological Research, Boston, November 1972.
44. Wikler, A. Requirements for extinction of relapse-facilitating variables in a narcotic antagonist treatment program. Paper presented at the First International Conference on Narcotic Antagonists, Warrenton, Virginia, November 1972.
45. Wikler, A. Annual Report, 1954, to Director, NIMH Addiction Research Center, Lexington, Ky.
46. Wikler, A., & Carter, R. L. Effects of single doses of N-allylnormorphine on hindlimb reflexes of chronic spinal dogs during cycles of morphine addiction. *J. Pharmacol. Exp. Ther.*, 109, 92-101, 1953.
47. Wikler, A., Fraser, H. F., & Isbell, H. N-allylnormorphine: effects of single doses and precipitation of acute "abstinence syndromes" during addiction to morphine, methadone or heroin in man (post-addicts). *J. Pharmacol. Exp. Ther.*, 109, 8-20, 1953.
48. Wikler, A., Martin, W. R., Pescor, F. T., & Eades, C. G. Factors regulating oral consumption of an opioid (etonitazene) by morphine-addicted rats. *Psychopharmacologia* (Berl.), 5, 55-76, 1963.
49. Wikler, A., & Pescor, F. T. Classical conditioning of a morphine abstinence phenomenon, reinforcement of opioid-drinking behavior and "relapse" in morphine-addicted rats. *Psychopharmacologia* (Berl.), 10, 255-284, 1967.
50. Wikler, A., & Pescor, F. T. Persistence of "relapse-tendencies" of rats previously made physically dependent on morphine. *Psychopharmacologia* (Berl.), 16, 375-384, 1970.
51. Wikler, A., Pescor, F. T., Miller, D., & Norrell, H. Persistent potency of a secondary (conditioned) reinforcer following withdrawal of morphine from physically dependent rats. *Psychopharmacologia* (Berl.), 20, 103-117, 1971.
52. Woods, J. H., & Schuster, C. R. Reinforcement properties of morphine, cocaine, and SPA as a function of unit dose. *Int. J. Addictions*, 3, 231-237, 1968.
53. Woods, S. C., Alexander, K. R., & Porte, D., Jr. Conditioned insulin secretion and hypoglycemia following repeated injections of tolbutamide in rats. *Endocrinology*, 90, 227-231, 1972.
54. Woods, S. C., Hutton, R. A., & Makous, W. Conditioned insulin secretion in the albino rat. *Proc. Soc. Exp. Biol. Med.* (N.Y.), 133, 964-968, 1970.

This lecture is dedicated to the memory of our esteemed colleague, Daniel H. Efron, M.D., Ph.D., who did so much for the scientific advancement of neuropsychopharmacology.

FACTORS INFLUENCING TOLERANCE TO AND DEPENDENCE ON NARCOTIC ANALGESICS[1]

Joseph Cochin
Boston University School of Medicine

Despite intensive and exhaustive experimental work over the past century, and more especially over the past 10 years, the phenomena of tolerance to and dependence on the narcotic analgesics are puzzling and intriguing. They have puzzled and intrigued pharmacologists for many years; although we have learned a great deal about tolerance and dependence, the mechanisms responsible for their initiation, maintenance, and loss still remain obscure.

Many hypotheses to explain tolerance to the effects of the narcotic analgesics have been proposed, and some have been demolished over the years. The most important ones include: (*a*) Altered metabolic disposition and/or differential distribution in the tolerant *vis-à-vis* the nontolerant animal; (*b*) prevention of access of drugs to the site of action; (*c*) occupation and saturation of these receptor sites, thus preventing access secondarily; (*d*) cellular adaptation, a term that is ill-defined and vague, and which may be biochemical or physiological; and finally, (*e*) some sort of change, also at the cellular level, that resembles an immune reaction or a reaction analogous to memory. The last is really a subclassification under cellular adaptation since it postulates a basic change at the cellular level that may be extremely profound.

None of these hypotheses or explanations has been fully satisfactory. For some, (e.g., prevention of access of the drug to the site of action), there is little or no evidence to indicate that such mechanisms play any significant role in the development of tolerance. Others, such as altered metabolism or differential distribution in the tolerant animal, have had much more widespread acceptance. This was especially true in the late 19th and early 20th century. Even when I

[1] Supported, in part, by NIMH grant MH 07230.

started working in the field some 25 years ago, this explanation was still the one generally held by most investigators. At the turn of the century, Marmé [27] proposed the conversion of morphine to an oxidized metabolite, a metabolite that was a stimulant whose action counteracted the depressant action of additional doses of morphine and whose action was uncovered when chronic administration of morphine was terminated, thus accounting for both tolerance and dependence. Since no such metabolite has ever been found, this theory is only of historical interest. It did anticipate, however, the "dual action" hypothesis of Tatum, Seevers, and Collins [36] and of Seevers and Woods [32] which formulated a neuropharmacological theory with a striking resemblance to the Marmé hypothesis, which was chemical in nature.

This concept that tolerance may be due to altered metabolism and/or distribution and excretion is an inviting one because evidence for it should be relatively easy to gather. It was one that until relatively recently most investigators held as a working hypothesis. In the past two decades, a large number of investigations would seem to have laid to rest theories of tolerance which invoke altered metabolism or disposition of chronically administered narcotic analgesics as an explanation of tolerance. Although I did my thesis problem at the University of Michigan using chemical methods to analyze tissues and biological fluids for morphine, the use of radioisotope and other more sophisticated techniques by others has not yielded any results contrary to our conclusions [8a] —namely, that neither the excretory pattern nor the tissues distribution is sufficiently altered in the tolerant animal to explain the many puzzling and sometimes incredible manifestations of tolerance.

Recently, Avram Goldstein [4] has suggested that both tolerance and dependence are completely and rapidly reversible and that tolerance, in part at least, can be explained by an increased rate of conjugation and excretion of the drug (levorphanol in this instance). The measure of drug effect in the mouse was an increase in activity after the administration of narcotic drugs. Rapid tolerance to this effect was noted. In our laboratory we have never seen the simple effect on activity that he describes, nor have we observed tolerance develop at anywhere near the same rate. We do see an initial depression of activity to which tolerance develops in a matter of days and a concomitant increase in activity which seemingly becomes even more marked as time goes on. This increased activity as drug administration continues is, we believe, more indirect since it is apparently due to the tolerance to the depressant effect of narcotics. In any case, the observations of Goldstein are extremely important if they can be replicated, and would be among the few that do not agree with the generally held conclusion mentioned earlier—namely, that altered distribution, metabolism, and excretion do not explain tolerance.

There are several explanations of tolerance on which I will not elaborate, since they do not really fit into the confines of my assigned topic or the space allotted, but I should mention in passing the receptor-occupation hypothesis, which was first postulated by Schmidt and Livingston [30] and which was based on their observation of acute tolerance to the vascular effect of morphine. This hypothesis assumed that drug molecules exert their action at the time of occupation of receptor sites and that, once attached, those drug molecules exert no effect other than preventing the initiation of a new response by receptor combination with additional drug. Although many aspects of morphine action are explained by this theory, there are facets of morphine action that point to much more profound changes. Among these are the persistence of tolerance and the appearance of abstinence symptoms long after the drug has apparently left the body. It is hard to visualize simple occupation of receptor sites for periods of several weeks, let alone the nine months to a year that tolerance has been shown to persist.

The idea that, based on biochemical changes, cellular adaptation may be one of the mechanisms of tolerance development is an intriguing one. Enzymatic adaptation is a well-known phenomenon in biology, and cytochemical studies have shown that the distribution and concentration of H^+, SH groups, nucleic acids in liver cells, and so on are affected by extrinsic factors such as diet and physiological condition of the animals. Such biochemical transformations may conceivably take the form of an increased or decreased activity of mechanisms normally operating to carry on a function, or may occur through the substitution of alternative pathways. The forms of such adaptations may differ from phenomenon to phenomenon and from preparation to preparation, but the term "adaptation" is broad enough to cover a wide range of changes that are responses to external stimuli and the external environment. Such changes are most often intracellular and can include alteration in levels of enzyme activity, in the respiration of cortical slices, in the reaction of offspring of mothers who were treated with drugs chronically before pregnancy, as well as the evoking of mechanisms to maintain homeostasis. These changes may also include the response of animals and man to drugs with reactions that resemble those seen in immunological processes and memory.

The theories invoking homeostatic adjustments to account for tolerance are quite old and although many of them cannot really be classified as biochemical, many can; and the resemblance between those that invoke biochemical adjustments in so many words and those that infer them is striking. There is, for instance, much in the "dual action" theory of Seevers and Woods [32] that anticipates in a neuropharmacological way the "derepressor" theories of Shuster [33], Goldstein and Goldstein [19] and Collier [13]. They all invoke homeostatic adjustments and stimulant and depressant effects existing side by side, but the former are covered by the latter and become unmasked during withdrawal. Thus, Marmé's [27] hypothesis mentioned earlier is an example of an ingenious unitary theory based on no evidence at all.

The dual action hypothesis postulated by Seevers and Woods [32] several decades ago is another example of the homeostatic adjustment hypothesis and was based on the postulate that depressant and stimulatory receptors for morphine are in different sites on or in the neuron, that the depressant action masks the stimulant action during the course of drug action, and that upon termination of drug administration the stimulant properties of morphine are unmasked and the withdrawal syndrome results. Despite the attractiveness of this formulation, recent experiments from the same laboratories at the University of Michigan lead us to the conclusion that it is not a valid explanation of the phenomena it attempted to elucidate [31].

Changes in enzymic activity with tolerance have long been postulated and looked for, but it was not until the classic studies of Axelrod [1] in the late 1950s that any meaningful correlation was made between enzymic activity and chronic morphine administration. He showed that an N-demethylase, one found in rat-liver microsomes, was able to N-demethylate such narcotic drug substrates. He also found that the pharmacologically active stereo isomers of many of the narcotic drugs were demethylated at much higher rates than the nonactive optical isomers. In addition, he and I found that nalorphine and other antagonists inhibited the in vitro N-demethylation of narcotic drugs but not of non-narcotic drug substrates [3]. In view of these similarities between the receptor sites for the narcotic analgesics and the N-dealkylating enzymes—stereospecificity, nalorphine inhibition, and substrate specificity—Axelrod decided to investigate the effect of chronic morphine administration on N-demethylase activity. He found that chronic administration of morphine depresses N-demethylase activity, that nalorphine given concomitantly with morphine blocks the enzyme depression to some extent, depending on the morphine-nalorphine ratio, that non-narcotic drug substrates were not affected by chronic administration of morphine, and that 12 days after withdrawal the demethylase activity has completely recovered. On the basis of these findings, he postulated that this enzyme system might serve as a model for the analgesic drug receptors and that changes in one paralleled changes in the other. He suggested that tolerance might be due to inactivation of receptor sites by their occupation by narcotic drugs. In a like manner, the continuous interaction of narcotic drugs with demethylating enzymes inactivated the enzymes, resulting in the profound depression of N-demethylation seen after chronic administration of narcotic drugs [2].

As a logical follow-up of this work, Axelrod and I [7] decided to measure simultaneously the biochemical and pharmacological changes involved. We gave morphine, nalorphine, and normorphine chronically to rats and measured both depression of N-dealkylase activity by these substances and the analgesic response to morphine during and after chronic administration of these substances. Our results showed that both parameters of drug action were affected in parallel fashion and were consistent with the hypothesis that the depression of N-dealkylation parallels a decrease in the number of available drug-receptor sites. We also showed that nalorphine was able to induce cross-tolerance to morphine—a surprising finding at a time when the agonist nature of nalorphine was not well understood.

Another finding of great interest was the ability of normorphine to depress N-dealkylation despite the fact that normorphine cannot serve as a substrate for an N-dealkylating enzyme since its nitrogen atom has no alkyl substituent on it.

If the depression of N-demethylation was simply a nonspecific exhaustion of an enzyme being challenged with more and more substrate, then normorphine should have no effect. If, on the other hand, there is some relationship between tolerance and the reduction of enzyme activity, one would expect an effect on this activity even though the compound producing tolerance is not a substrate. This turned out to be the case. There was moderate cross-tolerance to morphine and moderate reduction of N-demethylase. Both parameters were affected to about the same degree by normorphine and nalorphine and this seemed to be correlated with the degree of tolerance to morphine these compounds induce.

During the past decade, many studies have been undertaken to either support or disprove Axelrod's concept. In any case, even those who have disagreed strongly with his conclusion have emphasized that "this hypothesis has stimulated a tremendous amount of productive experimental research in an area that has been characterized by ill-defined concepts and untestable formulation [38]."

Much additional work has been done on the relationship of tolerance and microsomal enzyme systems. I found that the stereospecifity that was one of the major cornerstones of Axelrod's theory was a species-specific property rather than a potency-linked attribute, and that even in the rat some d- and l- isomers inhibit N-demethylation equally well, whereas the d- isomers are without activity *in vivo*. I also found that, although the depression of enzyme activity and the development of tolerance paralleled one another, the recovery of enzyme activity after withdrawal was much more rapid than was the recovery of drug sensitivity (Figure 1) [8].

Johannesson and coworkers [21] have also studied the time course of tolerance development and its relationship to enzymatic activity. They found, as I have, that tolerance to analgesia can be produced by just two or three low weekly doses of either morphine or codeine, whereas the drug-metabolizing enzymes are decreased only after more prolonged administration of the same amount of the two drugs. It seems evident that the relationship of the effect of chronic administration of the narcotic analgesics on N-dealkylation and on tolerance is complex and unresolved. Much of these contradictory and seemingly unrelated data concerning microsomal enzymes needs repeating and expanding, if only to establish that the observed changes are completely coincidental and not related to tolerance.

On the biochemical level, homeostasis is, as I have mentioned, invoked in the various "derepression" theories proposed by Shuster [33] and by Goldstein and Goldstein [19] at about the same time, and modified by Collier [13] several years later. Shuster cited the presence of derepressors in certain bacterial enzyme systems as an explanation of enzymic induction and stated that many examples of derepression can be gathered from the actions of mammalian enzymes, especially those metabolizing drugs and carcinogens. Some of the carcinogens that act as enzymic inducers or derepressors may do so by nature of their similarity to naturally occurring steroid repressors. There are also examples of

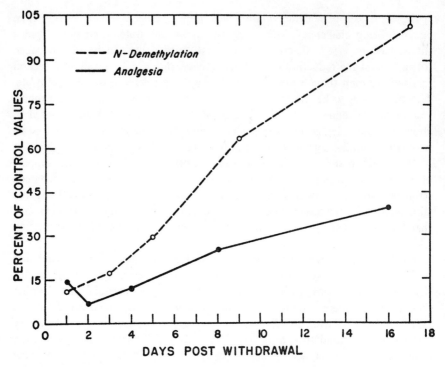

FIG. 1. Comparison of the recovery of drug sensitivity as measured by the hot-plate assay and liver *N*-demethylase activity in groups of chronically morphinized rats sacrificed at the indicated intervals after termination of drug administration. The ordinate is expressed as percent of values obtained in untreated controls. (*Adapted from Cochin and Economon [8].*)

drug-induced enzyme repression in the literature: One of the most striking is the marked decrease in microsomal *N*-demethylase activity, first described after chronic morphine administration by Axelrod [2], which I have discussed at length.

Theories of derepression all invoke inhibition of a hypothetical neurohormone that is responsible for selected CNS activity. Inhibition of the action of this hormone causes the depression characteristically seen after the administration of narcotic analgesics. The inhibition sets off a series of mechanisms that result in the overproduction of the neurohormones. The neurohormones neutralize the depressant effect of morphine and result in what we describe as tolerance. When morphine is withdrawn, the action of an increased amount of neurohormone is no longer antagonized or masked by morphine, and the result is the general stimulation of the CNS typically observed in abstinence. Collier [13] has modified this concept of Shuster's and of the Goldsteins. He proposes a receptor-induction theory in which more receptors for this hypothetical neurohormone become available with chronic administration of a narcotic drug.

Because more receptors are available, the number that combine with the neurohormone are maintained at a normal level and thus, despite continued depression of neurohormone levels by the drug, function remains normal. When the drug is withdrawn there is a large increase in the level of neurohormone, and the abstinence syndrome is seen.

All these hypotheses and attempts to consider tolerance and dependence as two sides of a single coin are in accord with biochemical theory. Unfortunately, the supporting experimental evidence is meager and inconclusive. All three hypotheses have as a common feature a neurohormone, the inhibition and overproduction of which triggers the development of tolerance. The evidence for the existence of such a compound or such compounds is slim despite exhaustive searches by Vogt [37], Maynert [29], Gunne [20], Martin [28], and others. Although some changes in catecholamine concentration during the addiction cycle have been found, none of these is large enough or temporally related in a convincing manner or sufficiently independent of other changes, such as stress, to allow one to postulate any causal relationship between catecholamines and/or precursors and tolerance and dependence.

An interesting relationship between the catecholamines and an effect of narcotic analgesics has been found by Smith [34, 35] in this country and by Weinstock [41, 42] in England. Both were studying the formations of lenticular opacities following the administration of opioids to mice and found a correlation between the rate of cataract induction and catecholamine administration; the higher the catecholamine dose, the lower the opioid dose necessary to produce cataracts. Thus, catecholamines are directly implicated in the formation of lenticular cataracts, and the development of tolerance to the opioid effects also affects the amount of epinephrine needed to potentiate cataract production. Tolerance to the lenticular effect developed very rapidly. Smith described two forms of tolerance—one that persisted up to 8 hours, and a second one detectable for at least 3 weeks. The short-term tolerance did not develop when small amounts of drug were given. On the other hand, the long-term type of tolerance was dose-related and could be detected with small doses of drug.

Within the past few years, Way and his associates [39, 40] have investigated changes in the rate of brain serotonin turnover during chronic administration and after abrupt withdrawal of morphine in mice. Although several people have reported unchanged levels of serotonin during chronic morphine administration, these measurements did not take into account the rate of serotonin synthesis in the brain—the turnover rate, in other words. Way determined the rate of serotonin synthesis and found that the turnover of serotonin in brain is markedly increased during the development of tolerance and then returns to normal within 2 weeks after discontinuation of morphine. He also found that the inhibition of serotonin synthesis with P-chlorophenylalanine markedly affected the development of tolerance in animals receiving morphine chronically and inhibited the development of physical dependence. At this time the relationship between serotonin turnover changes, tolerance, and dependence is not at all clear, but they may all be parts of closely related phenomena even though they may not be causally related.

Kornetsky and I, believing that a phenomenon must be adequately described before the mechanism of its development can be determined, initiated a series of experiments to characterize more precisely the development and loss of tolerance to morphine. In designing the experiments we took into consideration something that many investigators had either overlooked or ignored. In the very process of evaluating tolerance to morphine by giving animals a test dose of the drug, the phenomenon that one is attempting to measure is either initiated or made more profound. Thus each injection of morphine that is being used to test the development or loss of tolerance acts as a priming dose and changes the course of tolerance development and loss. To get around this difficulty we designed an experiment in which (using large numbers of experimental and control groups) the persistence of tolerance was studied in animals that had received morphine chronically and were then withdrawn; this was compared to the development and persistence of tolerance in animals that had received a single morphine injection or at most several injections at regular intervals. The results of such an experiment are shown in Figure 2 [9].

It is evident that a single injection of morphine given as long as 12 months earlier affected significantly the response to a second injection of the same dose of morphine. Animals that had received daily injections over a period of more than 2 months still showed decreased sensitivity to the morphine effect 15 months after their last previous morphine injection. Our results indicated that what is important in maintaining tolerance to morphine is not necessarily the length of the previous period of chronic morphine administration or even, within certain limits, the amounts given, but rather a history of a few previous injections of the drug—sometimes just one, depending on the interval. The results were consistent with those of Winter [44], who reported many years ago that the same degree of tolerance was induced by daily doses of morphine given to rats for 3 weeks, or bi-weekly injections for the same period of time. Similar findings have been reported in the mouse, with the tail-flick response to heat used as the measure of drug effect and several weeks as the elapsed time. Fraser and Isbell [16] also reported tolerance in man to the nauseant and emetic effect of morphine on body temperature 6 months after termination of chronic morphine administration. The comparisons were made with the effects of the drug on the same parameters in normal volunteers after a single injection.

Some years ago Eddy [14] noted that a second injection of morphine given to mice 24 hours following an initial dose did not seem to initiate the development of tolerance to the analgesic effect of the drug. However, if there was a 72- or 96-hour interval between the first and second injection, the effect of the second injection was attenuated. Recent work in my laboratory indicates quite clearly that the interval between injections is an extremely important factor in determining how much attenuation of effect results—another indication that the phenomenon of tolerance is a process requiring a finite amount of time for initiation and once instituted is amazingly persistent.

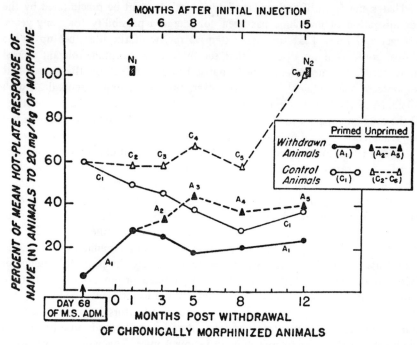

FIG. 2. A comparison of the response to 20 mg/kg of morphine sulfate of each of the animal groups on the hot-plate procedure at various intervals during the experiment. Animals in the primed group (closed or open circles) received injections at each point indicated. Each triangle (closed or open) represents a separate group of animals that were tested only once at the indicated interval. Groups N_1 and N_2 represent naive animals that were brought into the laboratory at the same time as the withdrawn and control animals but were never given morphine except at the indicated points. (*Cochin and Kornetsky [9].*)

With respect to the types of changes that might account for the persistence of tolerance up to 1 year after the last exposure of an animal to morphine and to other narcotic analgesics, most of the widely accepted explanations of tolerance have been found wanting. The possibility of the induction of a mechanism resembling an immune reaction is one that we found most inviting. It has been observed by many workers in the field of immunochemistry and immunology that the effects of a single previous dose of an antigen may be extremely long-lived, sometimes lasting for the lifetime of a given animal or man. Drug-induced antigen-antibody reactions are unfortunately not an uncommon occurrence, penicillin reactions being among the better-known examples. It has been suggested that tolerance, since it can be extremely persistent and since it does take time to develop, might be an immunelike phenomenon, a reaction to administration of a drug that was conditioned by the previous administration of the same drug or one closely related to it in structure or action.

That some form of antigen—antibody reaction might be precipitated by the administration of morphine has been considered a possibility for many years. Krueger and Eddy [25], in their extensive review of the literature up to the 1940s, could find no evidence that serum from a morphine-tolerant animal transferred to a nontolerant test animal had any effect on the subsequent response of the recipient animal. However, these early experiments dealt with tolerance to the lethal effect of morphine, and not with tolerance to the effect of the drug on behavior or on reaction to noxious stimuli, and may therefore not be germane.

In our laboratories, Kornetsky and I [10] conducted experiments involving transfer of serum from tolerant donors to nontolerant recipients to see whether there was a factor that could possibly be transferred. In preliminary studies, Kornetsky and Kiplinger [24] and Kiplinger and Clift [22] had found evidence of a factor in serum of tolerant dogs that potentiated, rather than attenuated, the action of morphine. We then attempted to see whether this factor was present in other species; we used rabbits and rats as donor animals, and mice as recipients. Our results, although inconclusive, indicate the possible presence of factors in the serum of tolerant animals that attenuate or potentiate the effect of morphine in recipient animals, depending on the experimental conditions and the species. In the past several years some investigators have described the transfer of factors from extracts of tolerant and nontolerant mouse brains that modified the response to morphine in recipient mice. This work has yet to be repeated, and the presence of such transferable factors has not yet been demonstrated conclusively.

Our more recent approaches to the problem of elucidating the nature of tolerance have been somewhat different. Kornetsky was interested in delineating the onset of tolerance after a single injection, and used as a measure of drug effect a modification of the voltage-attenuation technique first described by Weiss and Laties [43]. In this procedure an animal is put on a grid through which an electric shock can be delivered. The animal is then trained to press a lever or turn a wheel to attenuate the intensity of the shock to tolerable levels. After a no-drug baseline is obtained, morphine is administered, and the tolerated shock levels are then determined at specific intervals after drug. From the data obtained it is then possible to calculate the area under the time-response curve in a similar manner as in the hot-plate analgesic assay.

Figure 3 shows the results of an experiment using this technique. Each rat in the experimental group received 10 mg/kg of morphine on day 0 and a second injection of 5 mg/kg on the days indicated on the slide, and was then tested on the apparatus [23]. The mean scores of the 8 experimental animals were compared with the mean scores of 8 control rats that had never received morphine previously and that were given their first injection of morphine on the same test day as the experimental animals and tested on the attenuation apparatus. It is apparent even by day 3, and certainly by days 15 and 31, that the effects of a second injection of morphine are significantly diminished. The time course of tolerance is also of interest: it is significantly greater at 6 months than at 1 month. On the other hand, a second injection has no attenuating effect when given 24 hours after the first injection. The results, which agree with those observed by Eddy and others, are additional evidence that the tolerance phenomenon takes time to develop fully.

To better understand what the characteristics of tolerance are, we undertook to study in our laboratory and describe more fully the various factors that affect long-term persistence of drug effect, to help explain why tolerance develops more rapidly and more completely under some conditions than under others. We investigated the role that the interval between doses plays [11]. Rats were given 15 mg/kg injections of morphine and tested for their response to the drug. They were then divided into 3 groups which were given drugs at 1-week, 2-week, or 3-week intervals. The results, shown in Figure 4, were somewhat surprising. Animals receiving morphine at weekly intervals did not give responses significantly different from their initial reactions until the third injection, whereas the animals receiving morphine at 14- and 21-day intervals gave significantly diminished responses after the second injection. There are significant differences in response between groups until the fifth injection of morphine. Figure 5 shows the effect of intervals shorter than 7 days. It is almost as if the 7-day interval between doses were some sort of watershed—tolerance is induced more rapidly at longer and shorter intervals. It may be that the 7-day

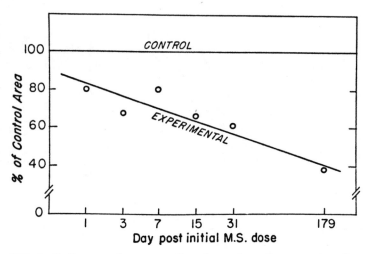

FIG. 3. Performance by rats on the voltage-attenuation apparatus after morphine. Animals in the control group received injections of 5 mg/kg on the designated days. Animals in the experimental groups received an injection of 10 mg/kg morphine sulfate on day 0 and an additional injection of 5 mg/kg morphine sulfate on one of the designated days. Each point represents eight control and eight experimental animals. (*Adapted from Kornetsky and Bain [23].*)

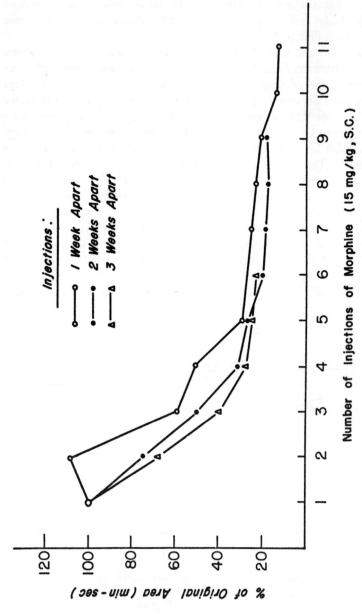

FIG. 4. The influence of intervals of 1 week or more on the development of tolerance to morphine. Injections of 15 mg/kg morphine sulfate were given at the indicated intervals. Animals were tested for their response to morphine using the hot-plate technique. The ordinate expresses percent of their original response. (*Presented in Cochin and Mushlin [11].*)

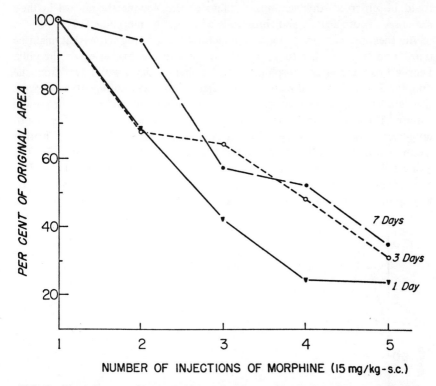

FIG. 5. The influence of intervals of 1 week or less on the development of tolerance to morphine. Injections of 15 mg/kg morphine sulfate were given at the indicated intervals. Animals were tested for their response to morphine using the hot-plate technique. The ordinate expresses percent of their original response. (*Cochin and Mushlin, unpublished observations.*)

interval marks the transition between long- and short-term tolerance, both of which have been described for morphine.

We have also studied the effects of concomitant injections of Freund's adjuvant with morphine [12]. Both pretreatment and concomitant administration alter the course of tolerance development. Figure 6 shows the effects of concomitant administration of morphine and adjuvant at weekly intervals. It is apparent that the development of tolerance is delayed by the administration of Freund's adjuvant at the same time. Figure 7 depicts the effect of pretreatment with adjuvant for 8 weeks followed by morphine administration. Here again potentiation of the morphine effect is shown, along with delay in tolerance development. The reasons for this seemingly opposite result to that expected remain obscure.

Since neonatal thymectomy profoundly alters immune responses in the rat, and reasoning that tolerance might be due to some immunelike mechanism, we hoped that such treatment would affect tolerance. No effect of thymectomy could be observed—thymectomized animals were completely normal in their responses to both acutely and chronically administered morphine [17].

Another approach was to look for a factor affecting drug action that might be transferred from mother to young across the placental barrier or via the milk. Female rats were given morphine for a number of days, withdrawn from the drug for 5 to 6 days, and mated to drug-free males. The resulting offspring were then studied for differences in sensitivity to drugs and differences in growth pattern. There were significant differences in weight between the offspring of drug-treated mothers and the offspring of controls, despite the fact that neither group of offspring was exposed to drug either *in utero* or *post partum* [18]. The greatest differences were found in the female young at 5-6 weeks of age. This experiment has now been repeated in mice, and there seems to be no doubt that very profound changes take place in animals treated chronically with the

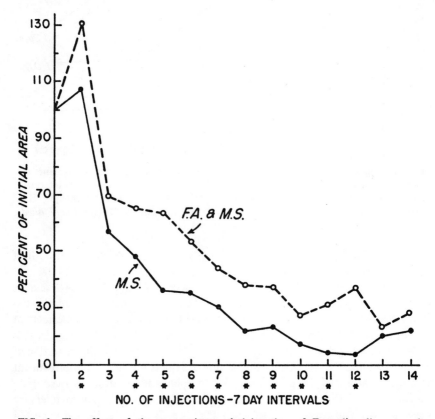

FIG. 6. The effect of the concomitant administration of Freund's adjuvant and morphine sulfate on the development of tolerance. Fifteen mg/kg morphine sulfate given at weekly intervals with or without 0.5 ml of Freund's adjuvant. Drug effect measured using the hot-plate assay. Ordinate measures percent of original area obtained after initial morphine injection. (*From Cochin and Mushlin [12].*)

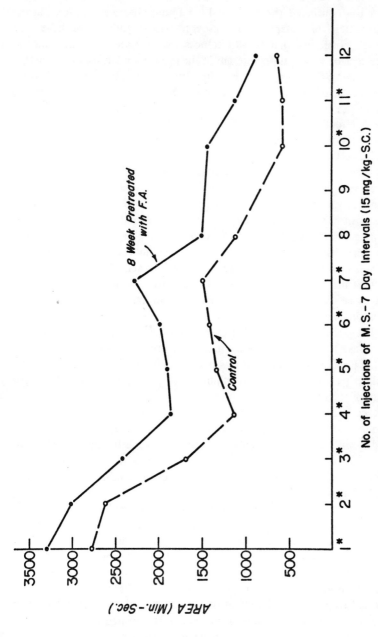

FIG. 7. The effect of 8-week pretreatment with Freund's adjuvant on the development of tolerance to a 15 mg/kg dose of morphine sulfate. The solid line represents the response of animals pretreated for 8 weeks with weekly injections of 0.5 ml of Freund's adjuvant, followed by weekly injections of 15 mg/kg of morphine. The dashed line represents the response of animals that received only morphine sulfate. The ordinate is the response obtained after the first injection of morphine sulfate. Drug effect measured by the hot-plate analgesic assay and expressed in units of area under the time-response curve. (*Cochin and Mushlin, unpublished observations.*)

narcotic analgesics, influencing—temporarily, at least—the developmental pattern of animals born 1 to 2 months after the last exposure of the mother to drugs. Dr. Friedler has continued the study and has found differences in mice in the second generation of offspring. By cross-fostering studies, we have also eliminated the possibility that the differences we have seen are due either to maternal neglect or to something present in the mother's milk. We do know that the factor affecting the young, whatever its nature, crosses the placental barrier. It is also possible, of course, that a profound disruption of endocrine balance may occur in the mother and that the chronic administration of morphine is thus indirectly affecting the growth of the neonate. It would, however, be difficult to explain effects of such a mechanism on second-generation offspring.

Obviously, effects so profound and long-lasting that they can affect succeeding generations must reflect long-lasting and profound cellular changes. At present, a number of laboratories, including ours, are attempting to modify these changes in various ways. A recent paper by Clouet [5, 6] describes a study in which she measured the incorporation of C^{14} into dopa, dopamine, and norepinephrine under conditions of acute and chronic morphine administration. She found that the accumulation of C^{14}-dopamine formed from injected C^{14}-tyrosine is increased in animals receiving morphine acutely, while in tolerant rats the rate of incorporation of carbon-14 into dopamine and norepinephrine is more than twice that seen after an acute dose of morphine in nontolerant animals. The incorporation into dopa, however, is less in tolerant animals. She interprets these results to suggest that protein synthesis is involved in tolerance for two reasons: first, after an initial inhibition protein synthesis is increased above normal levels in the brains of rats treated 24 hours earlier with morphine; and second, others have shown that inhibition of protein synthesis retards the development of tolerance.

We have carried out studies in our laboratories, as has Dr. Way in his, using cycloheximide, a potent suppressor of the synthesis of certain proteins and nucleic acids of memory and of immune reactions. Way has been able to show an increased sensitivity to a test dose of morphine and an effect on the development of physical dependence [26] after cycloheximide has been given to mice along with morphine.

In our laboratory we have attacked the problem somewhat differently. We have been interested, as I have mentioned, in the similarities between tolerance and immunelike or memorylike reactions—similarities which Kornetsky and I called attention to when we reported our first study of the long-term persistence of tolerance and of tolerance induced by a single previous injection [9]. We used cycloheximide because it had been used previously to disrupt memory traces, and we wished to determine the effect of the administration of cycloheximide when given an hour before the dose of morphine. We wanted to see whether it would affect the processes initiated by a morphine injection.

One of my students, Michael Feinberg, has carried out a series of experiments in which one group of rats was given single injections of 10 mg/kg of morphine

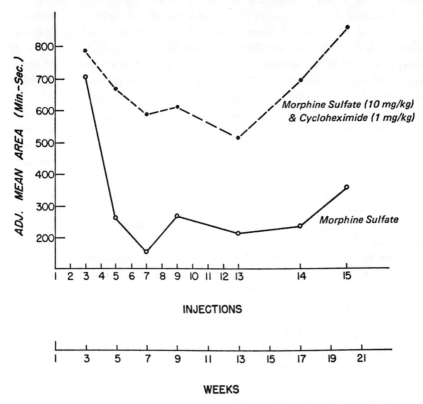

FIG. 8. The effect of the concomitant administration of morphine sulfate and cycloheximide on the development of tolerance as compared to the effect of morphine sulfate alone on the development of tolerance. Injections of 10 mg/kg of morphine sulfate were given 1 hour after the administration of 1 mg/kg of cycloheximide to those animals that received both agents. Injections of 10 mg/kg of morphine sulfate were given to those animals receiving only morphine sulfate. The animals were tested on the hot-plate for their response to morphine sulfate at each point indicated by either the closed or open circles. The ordinate indicates the adjusted mean area under the time-response curve. The abscissa indicates the schedule of injections and testing. *(Feinberg and Cochin [15].)*

every week for several weeks, while another group was given cycloheximide 1 hour before being injected with morphine [15]. All animals were then tested by the hot-plate analgesic assay technique. The results obtained are illustrated in Figure 8. There are striking differences between the two groups, and the development of tolerance is inhibited in animals treated with morphine plus cycloheximide. At week 13 the cycloheximide was discontinued for a period of 4 weeks, and the animals were tested for their response to a dose of morphine at week 17. As would be expected, the animals that received only morphine still showed almost complete loss of morphine sensitivity—a rapid loss of tolerance. By the 21st week, just 8 weeks after the last dose of cycloheximide, these animals had recovered sensitivity to morphine completely, whereas the morphine-alone group seemed to be as tolerant as at week 17. We have now expanded our experiments to include 6-hour and 24-hour pretreatment schedules with cycloheximide. Neither of these schedules seems to have any effect on tolerance development. If the morphine-plus-cycloheximide injections are given every other week and the results compared with those obtained from animals treated with cycloheximide in the intervening weeks as well, there are no significant differences between groups, but both groups are significantly different from morphine-only controls. It appears, therefore, that only the cycloheximide injections that are directly associated in time with the morphine injections have any influence on the consequences of the morphine injections.

I know that this cursory overview leaves more out than it includes, but the very complexity of the problem makes it impossible to clearly define and delimit its boundaries and ramifications. I have not even begun to consider the problems of drug-seeking, psychological dependence, and where it and physical dependence share a common ground. My hope is that this review will demonstrate very clearly how dependent clinical progress is on basic research. The treatment modalities that involve morphine antagonists and methadone could never have developed without the background and understanding that the laboratory research and the basic clinical studies at Lexington and other centers have contributed to our knowledge.

REFERENCES

1. Axelrod, J. The enzymatic N-demethylation of narcotic drugs. J. Pharmacol. Exp. Ther., 117, 330–332, 1956.
2. Axelrod, J. Possible mechanisms of tolerance to narcotic drugs. Science, 124, 263–264, 1956.
3. Axelrod, J., & Cochin, J. The inhibitory action of nalorphine on the enzymatic N-demethylation of narcotic drugs. J. Pharmacol. Exp. Ther., 121, 107, 1957.
4. Cheney, D. L., Goldstein, A., & Sheehan, P. Rate of development of reversibility of brain tolerance and physical dependence in mice treated with opiates. Fed. Proc., 29, 685, 1970.
5. Clouet, D. H. Protein and nucleic acid metabolism. In D. H. Clouet (Ed.), Narcotic drugs: Biochemical pharmacology. New York-London: Plenum Press, 1971.
6. Clouet, D. H. & Ratner, M. Catecholamine biosynthesis in brains of rats treated with morphine. Science, 168, 854, 1970.
7. Cochin, J., & Axelrod, J. Biochemical and pharmacological changes in the rat following chronic administration of morphine, nalorphine and normorphine. J. Pharmacol. Exp. Ther., 125, 105, 1959.
8. Cochin, J., & Economon, S. Recovery of N-demethylating activity and analgesic sensitivity in the rat following abrupt withdrawal of morphine. Fed. Proc., 18, 377, 1959.
8a. Cochin, J., Haggart, J., & Woods, L. A. Plasma levels, urinary and fecal excretion of morphine in non-tolerant and tolerant dogs. J. Pharmacol. Exp. Ther., 111, 74, 1954.

9. Cochin, J., & Kornetsky, C. Development and loss of tolerance to morphine in the rat after single and multiple injections. *J. Pharmacol. Exp. Ther.*, 167, 1, 1969.
10. Cochin, J., & Kornetsky, C. Factors in blood of morphine-tolerant animals that attenuate or enhance effects of morphine in nontolerant animals. In A. Wikler (Ed.), *Proceedings of the Ass ation for Research in Nervous and Mental Disease*. Vol. 46. *The Addictive States*. Baltimore: Williams & Wilkins, 1968.
11. Cochin, J., & Mushlin, B. E. The role of dose-interval in the development of tolerance to morphine. *Fed. Proc.*, 29, 685, 1970.
12. Cochin, J., & Mushlin, B. E. The effects of Freund's adjuvant on morphine sensitivity and tolerance. *Fed. Proc.*, 31, 528, 1972.
13. Collier, H. O. J. A general theory of the genesis of drug dependence by induction of receptors. *Nature* (London), 205, 181, 1965.
14. Eddy, N. B. The hot-plate method for measuring analgesic effect in mice. *Minutes of the 12th Meeting of the Committee on Problems of Drug Dependence*, NAS–NRC, *Appendix C*, 603, 1953.
15. Feinberg, M. P., & Cochin, J. Inhibition of development of tolerance to morphine by cycloheximide. *Biochem. Pharmacol.*, 21, 3082, 1972.
16. Fraser, H. F., & Isbell, H. Comparative effects of 20 mgm of morphine sulfate on nonaddicts and former morphine addicts. *J. Pharmacol. Exp. Ther.*, 105, 498, 1952.
17. Friedler, G., & Cochin, J. Sensitivity and tolerance to morphine sulfate (MS) in the rat as affected by neonatal thymectomy or MS-pretreatment of the mother. *Pharmacologist*, 10, 188, 1968.
18. Friedler, G., & Cochin, J. Growth retardation in offspring of female rats treated with morphine prior to conception. *Science*, 175, 654, 1972.
19. Goldstein, A., & Goldstein, D. B. Possible role of enzyme inhibition and repression in drug tolerance and addiction. *Biochem. Pharmacol.*, 8, 48, 1961.
20. Gunne, L. M. Catecholamines and S-hydroxytryptamine in morphine tolerance and withdrawal. *Acta Physiol. Scan.*, 58, Suppl. 204, 5, 1963.
21. Johannesson, L. A., Roger, J. R., & Woods, L. A. Tolerance to morphine and codeine analgesia and hepatic microsomal drug metabolism in the rat. *Acta Pharmacol. et Toxicl.*, 22, 255, 1965.
22. Kiplinger, G. F., & Clift, J. W. Pharmacological properties of morphine-potentiating serum obtained from morphine-tolerant dogs and men. *J. Pharmacol. Exp. Ther.*, 146, 139, 1964.
23. Kornetsky, C., & Bain, G. Single dose tolerance. *Pharmacologist*, 9, 219, 1967.
24. Kornetsky, C., & Kiplinger, G. F. Potentiation of an effect of morphine in the rat by sera from morphine-tolerant and abstinent dogs and monkeys. *Psychopharmacologia*, 4, 66, 1963.
25. Krueger, H., Eddy, N. B., & Sumwalt, M. *The pharmacology of opium alkaloids*. Pub. Health. Rep. Suppl. 165, 1941.
26. Loh, H. H., Shen, F. H., & Way, E. L. Inhibition of orphine tolerance and physical dependence and brain serotonin synthesis by cycloheximide. *Biochem. Pharmacol.*, 18, 2711, 1969.
27. Marmé, W. Untersuchungen zur Acuten und Chronischen Morphin Vergiftung. *Deut. Med. Wochschr.*, 9, 197, 1883.
28. Martin, W. R. Assessment of the dependence producing potentiality of narcotic analgesic. In L. Lasagna (Ed.), *International encyclopedia of pharmacology and therapeutics*. Vol. 1, Sec. 6. Glasgow: Pergamon, 1966.
29. Maynert, E. W., & Klingman, G. Tolerance to morphine. I. Effects on catecholamines in the brain and adrenal glands. *J. Pharmacol. Exp. Ther.*, 135, 285, 1962.
30. Schmidt, C. F., & Livingston, A. E. The relation of dosage to the development of tolerance to morphine in dogs. *J. Pharmacol. Ther.*, 47, 443, 1933.

31. Seevers, M. H., & Deneau, G. A critique of the "dual action" hypothesis of morphine physical dependence. *Arch. Internat. Pharmacolyn.*, **140**, 514, 1962.
32. Seevers, M. H., & Woods, L. A. The phenomena of tolerance. *Am. J. Med.*, **14**, 456, 1953.
33. Shuster, L. Repression and derepression of enzyme synthesis as a possible explanation of some aspects of drug action. *Nature* (London), **189**, 314, 1961.
34. Smith, A., Karmin, M., & Gavitt, J. Interaction of catecholamines with levorphanol and morphine in the mouse eye. *J. Pharmacol. Exp. Ther.*, **151**, 103, 1966.
35. Smith, A., Karmin, M., & Gavitt, J. Tolerance to the lenticular effects of opiates. *J. Pharmacol. Exp. Ther.*, **156**, 85, 1967.
36. Tatum, A. L., Seevers, M. H., & Collins, K. H. Morphine addiction and its physiological interpretation based on experimental evidences. *J. Pharmacol. Exp. Ther.*, **36**, 447, 1929.
37. Vogt, M. Concentration of sympathin in different parts of the CNS under normal conditions and after the administration of drugs. *J. Physiol.*, **123**, 451, 1954.
38. Way, E. L., & Adler, T. K. *The biologic disposition of morphine and its surrogates.* Geneva: World Health Organization, 1962.
39. Way, E. L., Loh, H. H., & Shen, F. H. Morphine tolerance, physical dependence and the synthesis of brain serotonin. *Science,* **162**, 1290, 1968.
40. Way, E. L., Loh, H. H., & Shen, F. H. Simultaneous quantitative assessment of morphine tolerance and physical dependence. *J. Pharmacol. Exp. Ther.*, **167**, 1, 1969.
41. Weinstock, M. Similarity between receptors responsible for the production of analgesia and lenticular opacity. *Brit. J. Pharmacol.*, **17**, 433, 1961.
42. Weinstock, M. & Stewart, H. C. Occurrence in rodents of reversible drug-induced opacities of the lens. *Brit. J. Opthalmol.*, **45**, 408, 1961.
43. Weiss, B., & Laties, V. G. Changes in pain tolerance and other behavior produced by salicylates. *J. Pharmacol. Exp. Ther.*, **131**, 120, 1961.
44. Winter, B. A. Measures of analgesic effect: The tail-flick method. *Minutes of the 12th Meeting on Problems of Drug Dependence*, NAS–NRC, *Appendix A*, 577, 1953.

RECENT RESEARCH ON OPIATE ADDICTION: REVIEW OF A NATIONAL PROGRAM

Stephen Szara
Center for Studies of Narcotic and Drug Abuse
National Institute of Mental Health

and

William E. Bunney, Jr.
Division of Narcotic Addiction and Drug Abuse
National Institute of Mental Health

INTRODUCTION

About a year ago the Division of Narcotic Addiction & Drug Abuse (DNADA) of the National Institute of Mental Health (NIMH) called together an *ad hoc* Advisory Committee of top researchers in the addiction area and the biomedical sciences (November 19, 1971, in Bethesda, Maryland) to help define the focus of an expanded research effort in the biomedical aspects of drug abuse. The biomedical area comprises about 50% of the NIMH research effort. In a large majority of the areas proposed for increased emphasis, a central concern was the pharmacological paradigm of tolerance and physical dependence.

RESEARCH FOCUS ON TOLERANCE AND PHYSICAL DEPENDENCE

Pharmacological tolerance to a drug and physical dependence on it can be operationally defined and readily lend themselves to further exploration through several research approaches.

They have been implicated as major physiological factors in the acquisition and maintenance of an opiate habit, especially heroin, with all the social and economic consequences that made the President declare drug abuse a major social problem in the United States. But the same paradigm has also served as a scientific basis to develop therapeutic approaches to treat the casualties of opiate dependence. What is even more important, however, is that the same paradigm may also serve as a guide to develop preventive measures for exposed and susceptible populations.

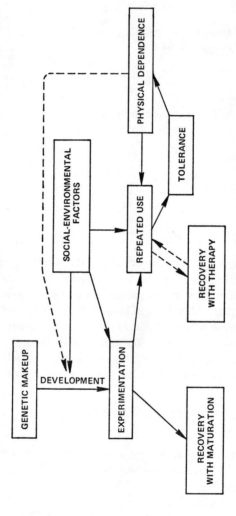

FIG. 1. Time course of events in opiate addiction.

The temporal course of events leading to the development of tolerance and physical dependence may be visualized, for our purposes, in a highly schematic way (Figure 1).

We have chosen to show that the genetic makeup of an individual may have an important role in determining the physical and psychological development of a person, and that experimentation with drugs may be considered a form of natural exploratory behavior. Whether or not exploration will include drugs will be largely determined by social-environmental factors such as availability, peer pressure, etc. Experimentation with opiates does not necessarily lead to dependence; as a matter of fact, a large number of youngsters will experiment a few times and then discontinue this type of behavior. Others may find the drug-produced euphoria desirable and continue opiate use. If opiates are used repeatedly at frequent intervals in sufficient doses, this will inevitably lead to the development of tolerance and physical dependence which tends to trap the individual in a vicious cycle. Several hypotheses have been proposed to explain the biochemical and physiological mechanisms involved in the development of tolerance and physical dependence. The various approaches will be discussed in some detail below. For the moment we would like to call attention to the relationships marked with dotted lines in Figure 1. The two arrows reciprocally connecting "Repeated use" with "Recovery with therapy" intend to suggest that complete recovery without relapse is the exception rather than the rule. This follows from the strong influence of social-environmental factors in causing the addict to relapse, in spite of the therapeutic efforts provided to break the vicious cycle of use-tolerance-dependence on opiates. Heroin addiction is often a recurrent illness.

The other broken line running from "Physical dependence" to "Development" suggests the possible important effect of narcotic addiction on the development of offspring of addicted mothers.

National Research Efforts

In order to place the research efforts sponsored by the NIMH into a national perspective, a few facts on federally supported drug research in fiscal year 1972 are reviewed.

The diagram in Figure 2 clearly shows that, although seven different federal agencies support drug-related studies, NIMH is responsible for supporting more than half of the federal program in terms of money spent for drug abuse research in fiscal year 1972.

NIMH Research Efforts

NIMH efforts in drug-related research are administered primarily by the DNADA and in FY 1972 amounted to a total of $17,241, most of which was channeled via grants rather than by contracts. In addition to this extramural

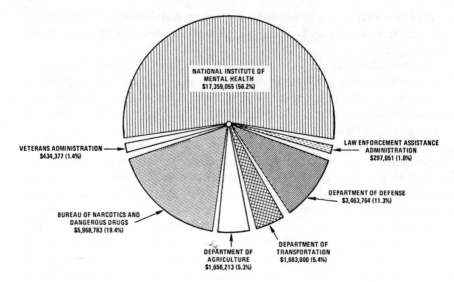

FIG. 2. Federally supported drug research for fiscal year 1972.

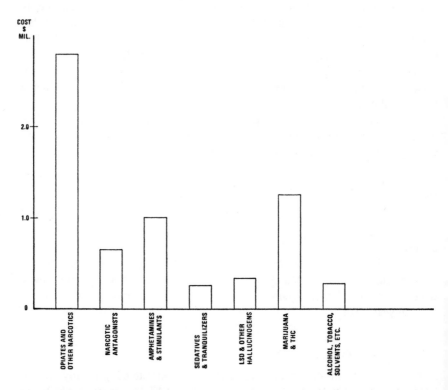

FIG. 3. Distribution of NIMH-supported drug research by drug class. Bars represent money spent for research on each class of drugs. The figures do not include grants channeled through the National Institute on Alcohol Abuse and Alcoholism.

research, the intramural effort at NIMH includes the Addiction Research Center in Lexington, Ky., with small components in the Bethesda and St. Elizabeths campus, and represents a relatively small portion of the total drug-related research efforts. Figure 3 shows an uneven distribution in grants, the largest mechanism by which NIMH supports drug research, in terms of class of drugs. By far the largest number of studies are concerned with opiates and other narcotics, with marijuana and THC occupying the second place, and amphetamines and stimulants the third.

The NIMH contract program deals almost exclusively with narcotic antagonists and marijuana-related research.

The distribution of the intramural program by drug category is somewhat similar to that of the extramural program.

RESEARCH TOPICS IN OPIATE ADDICTION

Because of our present focus on opiate-related research, we have broken down the opiate and narcotic antagonist grant support into seven areas according

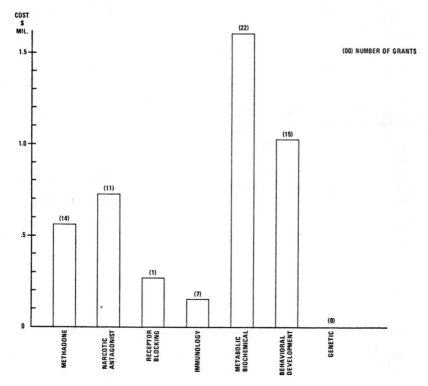

FIG. 4. Distribution of NIMH-supported drug research according to major emphasis on approach. Numbers at top of bars represent the number of grants supported during FY 1972, with total amount of money for whole program represented by height of column.

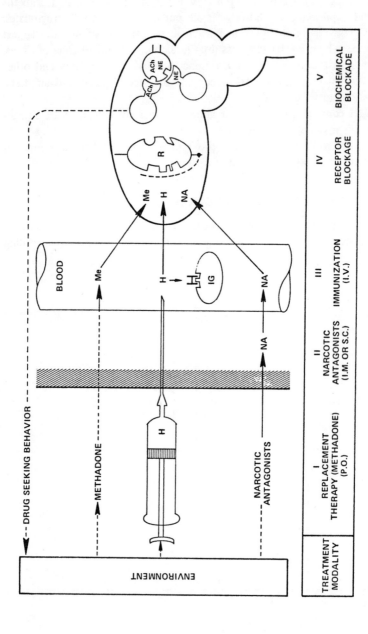

FIG. 5. Pharmacological approaches to treatment of opiate dependence. (ACh = Acetylocholine; H = Heroin; IG = Immunoglobulin; Me = Methadone; NA = Narcotic antagonists; NE = Norepinephrine; R = Receptor for opiates.)

48

to their potential implications for therapy and prevention of opiate addiction (Figure 4).

In the following summary we will review the rationales of seven therapeutic approaches based on the tolerance-dependence paradigm. Figure 5 respresents a visual conception of the five *pharmacological* approaches to treatment of opiate dependence. In addition, we will discuss the possible role of genetic factors in opiate dependence.

For the present discussion of research efforts in the five pharmacological categories, we shall assume that an opiate, most frequently heroin (H), when injected intravenously, reaches the brain via the blood stream partly unchanged and partly in the form of morphine to exert its typical euphorigenic effects by interacting with a hypothetical specific opiate receptor (R) in the central nervous system (CNS). The receptor is symbolized as having two allosteric sites: one for the opiates, the other for some endogenous substrate, as recently suggested by Goldstein [18]. Occupation of the receptor site is assumed to lead to biochemical changes, possibly involving neurotransmitters (symbolized by a synaptic arrangement on the right side of the diagram in Figure 5). The tolerance and physical dependence resulting from these biochemical changes together with the subjective experience of narcotic "high" are assumed to contribute significantly to drug-seeking behavior of the individual [44].

In reviewing the various pharmacological approaches, we shall mention the methadone maintenance therapy only briefly since it will be dealt with in detail by others in this book.

Methadone Maintenance Therapy

This therapy is based on the principle of cross-tolerance between methadone and opiate and on gradual accumulation of the drug followed by slow excretion. Orally administered methadone at a certain dosage level does not appear to have a euphorigenic effect but induces a marked, slowly developing tolerance to all opiate-like drugs, including methadone itself. As a result, the patient cannot feel the euphoric effect of ordinary doses of other narcotics such as heroin or morphine [12, 22].

Methadone maintenance treatment is viewed as a practical, although less than perfect, technological "shortcut" to the solution of the problem at hand [14, 25].

Although methadone maintenance has achieved a certain amount of success in moving the addict toward socially productive behavior, it has, since it is an agonist narcotic, also created medical and social problems such as diversion to illegal channels, overdose-related deaths, etc. [25]. These problems and possible ways of improving this treatment modality, such as the use of the longer-lasting 1-alpha-acetyl methadol (LAAM), are reviewed by other authors in this volume.

The NIMH is now supporting six grants on the chemistry, pharmacology, and toxicology of methadone and LAAM. We also support 11 grant programs for clinical research (in addition to the various treatment programs) with methadone and LAAM.

Narcotic Antagonist (NA) Therapy

NAs are drugs that are structurally similar enough to narcotics to occupy presumably the same receptor sites in the nervous system at which narcotics act, thus producing competitive inhibition as was reported by Takemori [38]. The main difference is that NAs have little or no agonistic (morphine-like) action at these sites, but by occupying them they prevent or reverse the action of the narcotics [15, 28].

The narcotic antagonists as a group are relatively free of abuse potential, and the risk of illicit redistribution is not a major limitation on their use, at least for the present.

Characteristics that seem to be important if a compound is to be useful as a narcotic antagonist in the treatment or prevention of addiction are: (1) ability to antagonize the euphoric high of opiates; (2) few or no pharmacologic effects of its own; (3) inability to cause physical dependence; (4) no evidence of increasing tolerance to its antagonistic actions; (5) absence of serious side effects and toxicity even in chronic use; (6) ease of administration; (7) long-lasting or moderate duration of antagonistic effects; (8) absent or low abuse potential; (9) reversible effects in case of medical emergency; (10) high potency, to permit administration of small amounts in a depot preparation; and (11) easy availability and low cost.

Since none of the antagonists available today meets all these criteria, the federal government has under way an intensive antagonist research program which includes three major elements: (1) preclinical research covering the synthesis of long-lasting antagonists to be used orally or as a depot preparation, screening for antagonistic activity in existing compounds, in-depth screening of selected compounds, and toxicity studies; (2) early clinical testing, including characterization of antagonist properties and pharmacological effects in man; (3) clinical efficacy studies evaluating patient acceptance, safety, and therapeutic efficacy.

The NIMH antagonist research program includes investigations at various institutions, universities, and medical schools, with grant and contract support. In addition, extensive work is being carried out at the NIMH Addiction Research Center in Lexington. The pharmaceutical industry is also involved in the search for and evaluation of antagonist chemicals. In addition, the Veterans Administration is now planning a large-scale multifacility clinical research program comparing antagonists to other forms of treatment.

Several chemically different antagonists are being tested. These include such drugs as cyclazocine, naloxone, EN1639A, l-BC 2605, and M 5050 (diprenorphine).

Two antagonists are already being used in experimental treatment programs: cyclazocine (a benzomorphan compound) and naloxone (N-allylnoroxymorphone), but they suffer the disadvantages of producing side effects in some addits or of being relatively short-acting.

Cyclazocine, which is the more widely used, in therapeutic doses will block both the habituating effects and the euphoria (or "high") from heroin for about 24 hours or more. In early treatment stages, patients may experience some unpleasant side effects unless their doses are built up gradually, but tolerance to these effects does develop [27].

Naloxone has far fewer side effects than cyclazocine. Pharmacologically, it is in some ways an almost perfect antagonist. It can be used to treat heroin overdose, with recovery from the effects of heroin beginning with a few minutes after naloxone injection. For the treatment and prevention of addiction, however, the drug is not ideal because its antagonist effects do not last as long as those of cyclazocine. The duration of action is short—from 4 to 10 hours. Further, naloxone is effective when given intravenously or subcutaneously, but requires huge quantities when taken orally.

Current research focus is on chemically modifying existing antagonist compounds to obtain forms that will act longer and be more potent and to develop preparations which have little or no side effects. Research investigators are also seeking to develop slow-release vehicles that would allow sustained action from a few days to a month [47].

Promising early results have been reported on research projects already under way in the development of new narcotic antagonists. One compound being studied is closely related to naloxone but appears to have some advantages over both naloxone and cyclazocine. The new drug Naltrexone (also known as EN 1639A) is 2 to 3 times more potent than both naloxone and cyclazocine, is effective orally, and has a longer duration of action than naloxone.

Even newer compounds were identified at the International Conference on Narcotic Antagonists jointly sponsored by the Center for Studies of Narcotic and Drug Abuse and SAODAP.[1] At least six of these compounds have enough pharmacological data to warrant further investigations.

The use of antagonists could be valuable in treating motivated patients, such as youths, who are not suitable subjects for methadone or related maintenance agents, or who have been addicted to heroin for only a relatively short time.

Narcotic antagonists could also be useful in a preventive role in the treatment of the casual user of heroin who has a high likelihood of becoming addicted. In the future, the prophylactic use of antagonists in high-risk areas may also be considered.

Immune Therapy

This approach is aimed at the possibility that specific circulating or mobilizable antibodies may bind injected heroin in the plasma and thus prevent the opiate from reaching the receptor site where it could be active.

Immunological concepts and techniques have contributed to biomedical research in opiate tolerance and dependence in three distinct areas:

1. Sensitive and specific immunoassays are being developed for the detection of opioids in the sera or urine of addicts. Some versions of these techniques,

[1] Special Action Office for Drug Abuse Prevention.

namely the hemagglutination-inhibition test of Adler and Liu [1], have reached the commercial markets, and sensitivity is already satisfactory since nanogram levels (1 ng/ml) in the urine or serum could be detected without extraction. However, work continues in various laboratories to increase the specificity of the technique. (We have two grants in this area.)

2. Several investigators have attempted to view the tolerance problem as an immunological phenomenon. Undoubtedly, there are several characteristics of tolerance to narcotic analgesics that resemble immunological phenomena, as Cochin pointed out [8, 9]. (Also see the Cochin chapter.) Among these are the persistence of some degree of tolerance for long periods after termination of drug administration even after a single dose of morphine; the fact that a definite period is needed to develop tolerance, and that the course of tolerance is affected by immunosuppressive agents and processes such as d-actinomycin, cycloheximide, and thymectomy. All these suggest the possibility that we may be dealing with an immunological process. However, as noted by Cochin, difficulties in attempting to transfer tolerance passively to nontolerant animals throw some doubt on this explanation, and the fact that most of the immunosuppressive agents are also nonspecific inhibitors of protein synthesis makes other interpretations of this phenomenon equally plausible. The phenomenon of cross-tolerance is also not explained. (We have three additional grants in this area.)

3. Morphine, by binding to a protein, can be made antigenic, and relatively specific antibodies can be produced, at least in animals, as shown by Spector and Parker [35]. This has raised hopes that a therapeutic approach to opiate addiction can be developed, using active immunization as a preventive measure. Several potential problems, however, will have to be solved before this therapeutic approach can be seriously entertained. Foremost is the question whether sufficiently high antibody titer can be obtained and whether anaphylactic reaction to injected morphine or heroin would not endanger the life of immunized subjects. Since there are several ways the morphine molecule could be bound to a protein and several different proteins possibly used to prepare these antigens [39], there is some hope that further research in this area may provide answers to the questions raised. Theoretically, at least, this could be developed into a new therapeutic approach to opiate addiction. (Again, we have two grants in this field.)

Receptor Blocking Therapy

While narcotic antagonists are acting in a reversible fashion, the antagonism being dependent upon the dynamic equilibrium between the antagonist molecules occupying the receptor site and those circulating in the blood stream, another potentially longer-lasting approach would be to try to inactivate or block the narcotic receptor sites by an irreversible inhibitor, which would not depend on continuously circulating molecules.

This approach is based on the concept of "affinity labeling" pioneered by Baker and his associates [2]. Active site-directed irreversible enzyme inhibitors have been applied recently to the analgesic receptor problem by Portoghese et al. [32] and May et al. [29].

Affinity labeling is an experimental procedure in which an appropriate synthetic derivative, usually an alkylating group attached to a specific substrate, is used *in vitro* or *in vivo* to irreversibly block a specific receptor site.

In the case of morphine, some preliminary *in vivo* animal data presented by Portoghese [32] suggest that this may be a profitable approach, but much more work is needed to develop it into a practical, therapeutic method. We also have one grant in which affinity labeling is being utilized in attempts to isolate and identify the hypothetical receptor for morphine [18, 45].

Biochemical Blockade Therapy

The rationale of this approach is based on the notion that a homeostatic balance of biochemical processes in the nervous system is disturbed by the chronic use of opiates which somehow represents the metabolic basis of tolerance.

We would probably have to make a distinction among biochemical processes underlying the psychological "high" and the ones which may be directly concerned with the genesis of tolerance and physical dependence. It is significant in this respect that the immediate pharmacological effects of morphine can be dissociated from those involved in the development of tolerance and dependence [3, 43]. In order to study this problem, increasing use is being made of newly developed techniques of selective destruction of central noradrenergic structures by 6-hydroxydopamine [16] and of central serotonergic structures by 5,6-dihydroxytryptamine [43].

Much work has been done to explore the role of neurotransmitters in mediating reward behavior in animals that may be considered a model for the psychological "high" or "rush." After the pioneering work by Olds [31] and Stein [36], a score of investigators explored the adrenergic hypothesis of reward mostly utilizing amphetamine as a stimulant, "reward"-producing drug (in the sense that it facilitates self-stimulation) [37]. Specific adrenergic blocking agents and specific enzyme inhibitors interfering with catecholamine metabolism have been used to test this hypothesis with controversial results [10, 46]. Whether or not the opiate-induced "high" or "rush" involves adrenergic mechanisms is controversial [16].

In regard to the biochemical basis for the development of tolerance, it is obvious from available experimental data that narcotic tolerance cannot be attributed to a change in distribution or an increased rate of metabolic inactivation of the opiate itself, as has been shown convincingly by Way and Adler [41]. It seems clear that the biochemical basis for narcotic action has to be sought not in the liver, where metabolic inactivation takes place, but in the central nervous system, where tolerance and physical dependence are most strongly expressed [30, 33].

What the nature of this biochemical disturbance is, and what its relationship has been to tolerance and dependence, is the subject of a great many investigations. There is little evidence that opiate-like drugs are interfering competitively with naturally occurring precursors of neurotransmitters in the CNS [13, 20]. The turnover of norepinephrine, dopamine, serotonin and/or acetylcholine can be affected by opiates in some species [42]; it may be the result of allosteric inhibition [18] and may be confined only to certain regions in the CNS [5, 24]. In addition, the complexity of the interrelationships among the neurotransmitters makes it difficult to ascribe a temporal primacy of drug action to any of the transmitters studied [3, 6].

In many of the hypotheses proposed to explain the biochemical bases of tolerance and dependence there is a requirement for the synthesis of macromolecules: either the synthesis of new molecules such as induction of the enzymes involved in neurotransmitter biosynthesis [19, 34], the synthesis of new receptors, increased protein synthesis following derepression of DNA by the opiate [7, 11], or a hypertrophy of redundant pathways [26]. Experimental evidence for these hypotheses is still mostly indirect.

Perhaps because of the challenging nature of these biochemical complexities, this is in many ways the liveliest area of narcotic research.

The numerous working hypotheses are being explored in the various laboratories, sometimes with intense commitments, creating occasional sparks and fireworks in professional meetings and on the pages of the scientific literature [4, 21]. This liveliness also shows up in the statistics of grants: NIMH is supporting 22 grants, among them several center grants whose focus is specifically directed at various aspects of the metabolic problems associated with opiate addiction. We have 9 grants which are concentrating on neurotransmitters and related enzymes, and 13 grants studying RNA and protein synthesis in broader terms.

Genetic Factors

A single or multiple genetic defect may be responsible for the synthesis of drug-metabolizing enzymes and may be the basis of an altered response to narcotic drugs. Pharmacologists are increasingly aware that some genes affect drug metabolism. A result of intensive investigations in pharmacology has been the emergence so far of some 10 inborn errors of metabolism affecting enzymes that biotransform drugs in man [40].

Long known have been the glucuronidation defects; others have been discovered recently [23]. Some of these errors are extremely rare; others are more prevalent. Some genetic defects lead drugs to cause uncommon adverse reaction; others may alter the intensity of the drug action [23].

How genes control drug action is becoming increasingly the subject of research because of our great progress in understanding the transmission of genetic information and because of new tools available for researchers. In FY 1973 we have one grant that proposes to investigate the genetic aspects of responses to opiates and other drugs, and two more to study evidence of chromosome aberrations in infants born to opiate-addicted mothers.

SUMMARY

The federal government is supporting a large, multimillion-dollar national program for research into the various aspects of drug abuse via seven of its departments coordinated by the Special Action Office. A large part of this program is channeled through NIMH, mostly via the grants and targeted research (contracts) mechanisms. Biological and pharmacological research on opiates and narcotic antagonists clearly represents an important focus in the total national effort in drug research. Tolerance and dependence are emerging as the foremost research paradigms around which several potential pharmacological therapeutic approaches are being built. Among these, the methadone maintenance and narcotic antagonist therapies are at the clinical stage of development and are providing admittedly partial answers to the narcotic addiction problems. Other approaches in the immunization, receptor blockade, biochemical blockade, and genetic directions are still at the preclinical research stage. The immediate goal of much of this research appears to be the identification of the opiate receptor and clarification of the role of biochemical changes underlying tolerance and dependence.

REFERENCES

1. Adler, F. L., & Liu, C. T. Detection of morphine by hemagglutination-inhibition. *J. Immunol.*, **106**, 1684–1685, 1971.
2. Baker, B. R. *Design of active site directed irreversible enzyme inhibitors.* New York: Wiley, 1967.
3. Bhargava, H. N., & Way, E. L. Acetylcholinesterase inhibition and morphine effects in morphine tolerant and dependent mice. *J.P.E.T.*, **183**, 31–40, 1972.
4. Cheney, D. L., & Costa, E. Narcotic tolerance and dependence and serotonin turnover, Technical Comments. *Science*, **178**, 647, 1972.
5. Cicero, T. J., Sharpe, L. G., Robins, E., & Grote, S. S. Regional distribution of tyrosine hydroxylase in rat brain. *J. Neurochem.*, 1973, in press.
6. Clouet, D. H. Theoretical biochemical mechanisms for drug dependence. In S.J. Mulé & H. Brill (Eds.), *Chemical and biological aspects of drug dependence*. Cleveland: CRC Press, 1972.
7. Clouet, D. H. Protein and nucleic acid metabolism. In D. H. Clouet (Ed.), *Narcotic drugs, Biochemical pharmacology*. New York: Plenum Press, 1971.
8. Cochin, J. Role of possible immune mechanisms in the development of tolerance. In D. H. Clouet (Ed.), *Narcotic drugs, Biochemical pharmacology*. New York: Plenum Press, 1971.
9. Cochin, J. Possible mechanisms in development of tolerance. *Fed. Proc.*, **29**, 19–27, 1970.
10. Corrodi, H. K., Fuxe, K., Hamberger, B., & Lynngdahl, A. Studies on central and peripheral noradrenaline neurons using a new dopamine-beta-hydroxylase inhibitor. *Eur. J. Pharmacol.*, **12**, 145–155, 1970.

11. Cox, B. M., & Osman, O. H. The role of protein synthesis inhibition in the prevention of morphine tolerance. *Brit. J. Pharmacol.*, **35**, 373, 1969.
12. Dole, V. P., & Nyswander, M. E. A medical treatment for diacetylmorphine (heroin) addiction, *JAMA*, **193**, 645-650, 1965.
13. Dole, V. P. Biochemistry of addiction. *Ann. Rev. Biochem.*, **39**, 821-840, 1970.
14. Etzioni, A., & Remp, R. Technological "shortcuts" to social change. *Science*, **175**, 31-38, 1972.
15. Freedman, A. M., Fink, M., Sharoff, R., & Zaks, A. Cyclazocine and methadone in narcotic addiction. *JAMA*, **202**, 191-194, 1967.
16. Friedler, G., Bhargava, H. N., Quock, R., & Way, E. L. The effects of 6-hydroxy-dopamine on morphine tolerance and physical dependence. *J.P.E.T.*, **183**, 49-55, 1972.
17. Fujimoto, J. M., & Haarstad, V. B. The isolation of morphine ethereal sulfate from the urine of the chicken and cat. *J.P.E.T.*, **165**, 45-51, 1969.
18. Goldstein, A. Interactions of narcotic antagonists with receptor sites. *Proceedings of the 1st International Conference on Narcotic Antagonists*, Airlie House, Va., November 1972. In press.
19. Goldstein, D. B., & Goldstein, A. *Biochem. Pharmacol.*, **8**, 48, 1961.
20. Harris, L. S. Central neurohumoral systems involved with narcotic agonists and antagonists. *Fed. Proc.*, **29**, 28-32, 1970.
21. Hitzemann, R. J., Ho, I. K., & Loh, H. H. Narcotic tolerance and dependence and serotonin turnover. *Science*, **178**, 645-647, 1972.
22. Jaffe, J. H. Research on newer methods of treatment of drug dependent individuals in the USA. *Proceedings of the 5th International Congress of CINP*, Amsterdam, Excerpta Medica International Congress Series **129**, 271-276, 1966.
23. Kalow, W. Genes controlling drug action in man. *5th International Congress on Pharmacology*, San Francisco, July 1972. Abstract, pp. 10-11.
24. Knapp, S., & Mandell, A. J. Narcotic drugs, effects on the serotonin biosynthetic systems of the brain. *Science*, **177**, 1209, 1972.
25. Lennard, H., Epstein, L. F., & Rosenthal, M. S. The methadone illusion. *Science*, **176**, 881-884, 1972.
26. Martin, W. R., Pharmacological redundancy as an adaptive mechanism in the central nervous system. *Fed. Proc.*, **29**, 13-18, 1970.
27. Martin, W. R., Gorodetzky, C. W., & McClane, T. K. An experimental study in the treatment of narcotic addicts with cyclazocine. *Clin. Pharmacol. Ther.*, **7**, 455-465, 1966.
28. Martin, W. R. Opioid antagonists. *Pharmacol. Rev.*, **19**, 463-521, 1967.
29. May, M., Czoncha, L., Garrison, D. R., & Triggle, D. J. The analgesic, hypothermic and depressant activities of some N-substituted α- 5,9-dimethyl-6,7-benzomorphans. *J. Pharm. Sci.*, **57**, 884-887, 1968.
30. Mulé, S. J. Effect of morphine and nalorphine on brain phospholipid metabolism. In A. Wikler (Ed.), *The addictive states*. Baltimore: Williams & Wilkins, 1968.
31. Olds, J. Hypothalamic substrates of reward. *Physiol. Revs.*, **42**, 554-604, 1962.
32. Portoghese, P. S., Telang, V. G., Takemori, A. E., & Hayashi, G. Potential nonequilibrium analgetic receptor inactivators, synthesis and biological activities of N-acylanileridines. *J. Med. Chem.*, **14**, 144-148, 1971.
33. Schuster, L. Tolerance and physical dependence. In D. H. Clouet (Ed.), *Narcotic drugs, Biochemical pharmacology*. New York: Plenum Press, 1971.
34. Schuster, L. *Nature*, **189**, 314, 1961.
35. Spector, S., & Parker, C. W. *Science*, **168**, 1347, 1970.
36. Stein, L. Effects and interactions of imipramine, chlorpromazine, reserpine and amphetamine on self stimulation: Possible neurophysiological basis of depression. In

J. Wortis (Ed.), *Recent advances in biological psychiatry*, Vol. 4. New York: Plenum Press, 1962.
37. Stein, L. Chemistry of reward and punishment. In D. H. Efron (Ed.), *Psychopharmacology, A review of progress, 1957-1967*. Washington, D.C.: U.S. Government Printing Office, 1968.
38. Takemori, A. E. The use of narcotic antagonists to characterize analgesic receptors. *Proceedings of the 1st International Conference on Narcotic Antagonists*, in press 1973.
39. Van Vunakis, H., Wasserman, E., & Levine, L. J. Specificities of antibodies to morphine, *J.P.E.T.*, **180**, 514, 1972.
40. Vesell, E. S. Pharmacogenetics, Introduction: Genetic and environmental factors affecting drug response in man, *Fed. Proc.*, **31**, 1253-1269.
41. Way, E. L., & Adler, T. K. *Bull., W.H.O.*, **25**, 227-262, 1961; **26**, 51-66, 1962; **26**, 261-284, 1962; **27**, 359-394, 1962.
42. Way, E. L., & Shen, F. H. Catecholamines and 5-hydroxytryptamine. In D. H. Clouet (Ed.), *Narcotic drugs, biochemical pharmacology*. New York: Plenum Press, 1971.
43. Way, E. L. Personal communication, 1972.
44. Wikler, A. Sources of reinforcement for drug-using behavior: A theoretical formulation. *5th International Congress on Pharmacology*, San Francisco, July 1972, abstract, 135-136.
45. Winter, B. A., & Goldstein, A. An arylazido analogue of levorphanol for the photochemical labeling of the opiate receptor. *Fed. Proc.*, **31**, A528, 1972.
46. Wise, C. D., & Stein, L. Amphetamine: Facilitation of behavior by augmented release of norepinephrine from the medial forebrain bundle. In E. Costa & S. Garattini (Eds.), *Amphetamines and related compounds*. New York: Raven Press, 1970.
47. Yolles, S. Development of long-acting delivery systems for narcotic antagonists. *Proceedings of the 1st International Conference on Narcotic Antagonists*. In press.

SECTION 2
INTRODUCTION

Conan Kornetsky
Boston University School of Medicine

Three of the following four papers review different approaches to the study of the narcotic analgesics. Two are concerned with psychological factors, while the third reviews some of the biochemical aspects of morphine dependence. The fourth paper by David F. Musto highlights how attitudes and social policy influence the research that is being done in the field of addiction. Although there is no underlying common theme in these four papers, they do clearly point out avenues for research with the narcotic analgesics and the manner in which research, at least in the past, has been influenced by public policy.

The first paper by Donald Overton is a review of the phenomenon of state-dependent learning (SDL) and the possible role that this phenomenon may play in the abuse potential of a drug. One of the characteristics of SDL is the discriminability of one drug from other drugs or even the discrimination of different doses of the same drug. Overton, in reviewing the field, finds a reasonable relationship between drug discriminability and abuse. In a table, he roughly rank-orders the discriminability of a variety of agents. Unfortunately, morphine is not among the highest; however, he does indicate that there is a paucity of data on the narcotic analgesics in this field. He presents a number of interesting theories to explain this rough relationship and suggests areas of research that will elucidate the role of SDL in abuse of drugs.

Schuster and Johnson systematically review for us several variables that contribute to self-maintained drug use, i.e., reinforcement variables, antecedent conditions, organismic variables, etc. For each of these variables, the review of the available literature offers a relatively complete picture of the present state of the art. Since the first report by Weeks in 1962 in *Science*, a number of laboratories around the country have used the technique of behavioral analysis of opiate dependence. At its simplest level, the procedure allows us to determine which drugs will sustain drug-seeking behavior; however, at its most sophisticated level, it allows for an experimental analysis of these variables that are relevant in maintaining drug-seeking behavior. The technique has broad implications for a rational understanding of drug-seeking behavior in man.

The third paper in the group is a marked change of pace. David Musto reviews the social and political influences on research in addiction. He focuses on the first quarter-century, with emphasis on the period just prior to and after 1920. It is clear in retrospect that the public and official attitudes markedly altered the type of research and treatment programs. Although the paper says nothing about the current scene, it is clear, at least to me, that there are currently attitudes prevalent in communities where drug abuse incidence is high and policies at the level of those responsible for public postures that have marked effects on the problems being investigated by scientists. It is unfortunate that research in drug abuse is shaped by such attitudes and policies; however, I doubt that anyone would be surprised to find similar influences in other areas of scientific investigation, especially if the research has broad implications to the various interest groups concerned with the handling of the problem.

The final paper by Way takes us back to the laboratory, but not the laboratory of the behavioral scientist as exemplified in the first two papers. Way brings us face to face with the fact that opiates cause profound changes in the biochemical milieu of the subject. Way reviews various types of pharmacologic manipulations that can modify the development of tolerance and physical dependence to the opiate drugs. He concludes from his experimental studies that it should be possible to use pharmacological agents to block the development of tolerance and physical dependence without altering analgesic efficacy. At the present time agents that will do this are much too toxic for human use. He further argues that if this could be done it would probably modify euphoria-producing effects of the drug and thus cause a decrease in compulsive drug use. A difficulty that I have with this concept is my belief that a great deal of the analgesic action of opiates may be intricately tied to what Way calls "euphoria." This euphoria that patients report may be related to the reduction-of-anxiety (over pain) properties of morphine, which I believe are an important component of the drug's analgesic action. Although Way's paper is concerned with the biochemical aspects of opiates, there are behavioral techniques used by Way and other biochemical pharmacologists. It is unfortunate that we could not in some way combine the sophisticated chemistry of Way with the sophisticated behavioral procedures discussed in the first two papers.

STATE-DEPENDENT LEARNING PRODUCED BY ADDICTING DRUGS[1]

Donald A. Overton

Eastern Pennsylvania Psychiatric Institute
and
Temple University Medical School

Available evidence increasingly supports the generalization that state-dependent learning (SDL) is produced by most abused drugs. This suggests that studies of SDL may predict the abuse potential of drugs, and also raises the possiblity that SDL may be causally involved in the addictive process. Although no explicit relationship between drug abuse and SDL has been demonstrated, experimental studies of this question have only recently begun. This paper will selectively review data on SDL which appear related to drug abuse, and will summarize the major theoretical formulations which have been put forward relating SDL to abuse.

SDL is said to occur if performance of a learned response is conditional upon the drug state present when the response was learned; i.e., if impaired performance results from any difference between the training and testing drug states. This is often tested by use of a 2 X 2 design in which four groups of subjects are trained and subsequently tested for recall in the states *N-N*, *N-D*, *D-N*, and *D-D*, respectively (*N* = no drug, *D* = drug). SDL studies using human subjects have been recently reviewed [39], although subsequent reports have appeared [22, 29, 56]. There has been no comprehensive review of SDL studies using animal subjects since 1967 [35], and many such studies have recently appeared. However, the methodological and interpretive difficulties associated with these studies are severe [40] and preclude any attempt to relate most of them to drug abuse at this time.

Studies using drug discrimination techniques have produced more consistent and interpretable results, and available data indicate that such discriminations

[1] Supported in part by NIMH grant 5-T02-MH05930-21.

are based on the same drug effects that produce SDL [32]. In such studies, rats are explicitly trained to perform one response in one drug state (e.g., right turn in a T-maze) and a second response (left turn) in another drug state. These studies have been recently reviewed in respect to alcoholism [39], and will be the primary data considered here.

REVIEW OF DATA

Properties of Drug Discriminability

Data from drug discrimination experiments appear to justify the following generalizations regarding the properties of drug discriminations.

1. If subjects are required to discriminate various doses of a drug from the no-drug condition, the discrimination is more rapidly acquired by the subjects given higher doses. Apparently discriminability is proportional to dose. This holds for all drugs tested with the exception of antimuscarinics, where both drug-state discriminability and various other CNS effects appear to asymptote at moderately high dose levels [37, 38, 57]. The degree of dissociation separating drug learning from no-drug learning is often inferred from the rapidity with which animals learn such drug versus no-drug discriminations [32].

2. Rats can differentiate between different doses of a single drug. The drug versus no-drug discrimination appears to be a special case of this ability to distinguish different dose levels [36].

3. The time course of drug discriminability appears to parallel that of other obvious CNS effects, such as ataxia [39]. Apparently the drug state present at the time of the learning experience determines the conditions for optimal recall, although it has been suggested that learning may be state-dependent if drug is administered immediately after training [24, 42].

4. After a rat is trained to differentiate a particular drug from the no-drug condition, it will tend to make drug choices during test trials with a variety of similar drugs, but not when tested with dissimilar drugs. It is difficult or impossible to train rats to differentiate between similar drugs if equally effective doses are used [18, 33].

5. Centrally acting drugs may be classified as similar or dissimilar on the basis of data from test trials and drug versus drug training [33, 40]. About a dozen discriminable (dissimilar) states are produced by administration of the various types of drugs shown in Table 1. Drugs of each class apparently produce states from which learning transfers only with a decrement to either the no-drug state or to the drug states induced by drugs in other classes. Rats may be trained to differentiate between dissimilar drugs [33].

6. Drugs which act only outside the central nervous system usually do not provide an adequate basis for rapidly acquired differential responding [18, 32, 33, 38].

7. Drug discriminations can often be established more rapidly than most

sensory discriminations [25, 32, 38]. This suggests that the formal similarities between drug discriminations and sensory discriminations may be more misleading than informative. In some studies there is no evidence to suggest that learning a drug discrimination actually involves discriminating the sensory consequences of drug action [7, 32]. Instead, differential responding appears to be based on the dissociative barrier which impairs transfer of training between the drug and no-drug conditions. However, in other studies using lower doses and operant tasks, the data suggest a more complex learning process which changes the shape of any preexisting dissociative barriers [54].

8. The ability to learn drug discriminations is not yet known to be restricted to any particular species or age group. Such discriminations have been reported with rats, cats, dogs, and monkeys [7, 15, 24, 38].

9. Drug discriminations can be obtained in a variety of behavioral tasks. The general characteristics of the phenomenon do not appear to vary as a function of the task selected [38], although the relative discriminability of different drugs may vary from task to task [54].

10. There is no evidence to indicate whether tolerance to the discriminable effects of drugs parallels tolerance to other drug effects. Using THC, Bueno showed that some discriminability persisted in rats which were substantially tolerant to the drug, but the study provided no data as to whether discriminability was reduced or unaffected by tolerance [9].

11. Drugs that are not easily differentiated from the no-drug condition are not subject to abuse. Conversely, most readily discriminable drugs are abused [38, 39]. It is this correlation which leads to our interest in the relationship of discriminability to abuse.

Relative Discriminability of Different Drugs

In order to rigorously compare the discriminability of various drugs, several requirements must be met: (a) A drug discrimination task must be used that is relatively insensitive to drug effects other than SDL, and in which the degree of discriminability can be quantified. (b) A decision must be reached regarding the dosage of each drug at which to compare discriminability. In practice, this might be accomplished by using some other task which gives a measure of overall behavioral toxicity. (c) The discriminability of each drug must be determined at the selected dose. A good way to do this is to obtain a dose response curve for discriminability, and derive from it an estimate for discriminability at the selected dose. On the basis of such procedures, one could reasonably compare the discriminability of various types of drugs and relate this to their respective abuse potentials.

The data now available fall short of these requirements in several respects: (a) Many different drug discrimination tasks have been employed. A T-maze task is often used, but performance may be motivated by electrical shock [32], hunger [2], or water escape [19]. Other varieties of shock escape tasks involving multiple alleys [34] or compartments [51] have also been used. Operant bar-pressing tasks are commonly used; these may involve two bars, one for each drug state [21], or two different reinforcement schedules on the same bar [1, 4, 18]. Both discriminated approach [27] and approach/avoidance tasks have been used [3]. Quantitative comparisons between measurements of drug discriminability made in these various tasks are not possible. (b) No measure of behavioral toxicity has been obtained which would allow us to select the dosages at which discriminability of various drugs is to be compared. (c) Most drugs have been studied at only a single dosage, and dose response curves have not been obtained. In practice, doses are usually selected so as to not produce excessive behavioral toxicity in the particular drug discrimination task employed. The sensitivity of these tasks to behaviorally toxic effects varies, leading different investigators to use different doses, even when studying the same drug.

Despite these difficulties, Table 1 is an attempt to rank-order a number of different types of drugs on the basis of their discriminability. The rank-ordering is primarily based on data obtained in the T-maze shock escape task. However, some of the drugs have been tested only in bar-pressing tasks, and the relative discriminability of such drugs has been estimated by comparision to drugs such as alcohol which have been tested in both T-maze and bar-pressing tasks. All in all, Table 1 should be regarded as more artistic than quantitative. Nontheless, this is the best that can be done with currently available data, and it seemed worthwhile to organize such information in this form.

The drugs tested for discriminability are listed in the first column in Table 1. These are arranged according to pharmacological classes. Generally speaking, pharmacologically similar drugs tend to be interchangeable in their discriminable effects, whereas dissimilar drugs are not interchangeable. However, recent research reveals added complexities as appreciable interchangeability often occurs between pharmacologically dissimilar drugs [4, 33, 40], and complete interchangeability within classes is not always found [4, 49].

The second column in Table 1 shows the dose or range of doses at which drug discriminability has been studied. Single-dose entries indicate that discriminability has only been tested at that single dose; in actuality, there is a range of probably effective doses. However, since the slopes of the dose response curves for various drugs differ [38], it is not possible to estimate the range of effective doses from measurements made at only a single or a few adjacent dosages. For some drugs, the lower end of the listed range is the lowest dose that has been studied. For more carefully studied drugs, a dose has been selected at which discriminability is approximately an order of magnitude less than at the maximum tested dose. The high end of the listed range of doses is generally a dose beyond which physical or behavioral toxicity prevents training in the shock escape T-maze task.

The third column in Table 1 lists sessions to criterion (STC) in the T-maze task for several drugs. More exactly, the STC column shows the geometric mean of the number of training sessions to begin criterion performance, where criterion performance is 8 correct first trial choices on 10 consecutive training

TABLE 1

Centrally Acting Drugs Tested for Discriminative Control

Drug	Doses	STC	N	References
Anesthetics				
Pentobarbital	10-20	1.3	16	3, 7, 11, 20, 32, 33, 36, 42
Phenobarbital	60-80	1.3	6	33
Secobarbital	15-20			33
Sodium barbital	150	3.3	3	33
Amobarbital	20-30			3, 33
Ethyl alcohol	1000-3000	2.6	6	1, 2, 3, 4, 12, 26, 27, 39
Meprobamate	200	2.4	12	3, 33
Paraldehyde	300			33
Ethyl carbamate	750	2.3	11	33
Chloral hydrate	200			3, 33
Hydroxydione	25			52
Progesterone	125			52
Ether				33
Nitrous oxide				
Benzodiazepines				
Librium	10-30	4.4	11	3, 4, 8, 18
Nicotinics				
Lobeline	40			37, 49
Nicotine	.4-4	2.8	14	30, 37, 40, 44, 45, 49, 50
Dissociative anesthetics				
Ketamine	10-60	5.5	9	40
Sernylan	5-20	7.1	6	
Antimuscarinics				
Atropine	5-200	4.4	18	4, 18, 26, 33, 34
Scopolamine	.2-300	5.3	12	33, 37, 38
Benactyzine	2-50	6.7	19	37, 38
Ditran	1-60	5.1	9	37, 38
Tetrahydrocannabinols				
Delta-9 THC	4-16			4, 19, 28
Delta-3 THC	4			4
Marijuana extract				4, 9, 28
Narcotics				
Morphine	9-36	12	3	20
Hallucinogens				
Mescaline	10-50	20	2	21, 48
LSD	.01-.1			48
Psilocybin	.4-2.5			18, 48

TABLE 1 (*Continued*)
Centrally Acting Drugs Tested for Discriminative Control

Drug	Doses	STC	N	References
Stimulants				
Amphetamine	.5-5	20	5	16, 18, 25, 54
Methylphenidate	4			17, 18
Convulsants				
Metrazol	30	10	3	
Bemegride	7.5	>22	6	33
Antinicotinics				
Mecamylamine	10-30	10	3	30, 37
Muscarinics				
Physostigmine	1	22	6	30, 33
Arecoline	1-10	34	6	46, 47
Carbacol	0.8	17	3	
Phenothiazines				
Chlorpromazine	4	>20	6	18, 33, 51
Acepromazine	8			51
Perphenazine	5			51
Prothipendyl	12			51
Dibenzazepines				
Imipramine	20-40	>20	6	33, 51
Virtually inactive drugs				
Pryilamine	50	>30	2	
Phenoxybenzamine	10	>50	3	
Caffeine	50	>60	3	
Aspirin	400	>60	2	
Lithium	80	>35	3	

NOTES:—Doses are mg/kg IP. in the rat. STC = geometric mean sessions to criterion.
N = number of rats averaged for STC. For $N < 6$, STC accuracy is low.

sessions. Column 4 shows the number of animals trained to obtain each STC value. The task has been described in more detail elsewhere [33, 37, 40]. Basically, rats receive a series of training sessions in which the imposed drug state and the required choice alternate so that one response is correct without drug and the other with drug. The dose used to obtain the STC value is the highest dose shown in the range of tested doses for all drugs except antimuscarinics, where minimal STC values are obtained with lower doses. Hence the value in the STC column reflects the most rapid discrimination learning which has been observed with each drug in the T-maze. In most cases the dosage is essentially the highest compatible with T-maze performance, with further dose increases being impractical due to either physical or behavioral toxicity.

The reader will note that drugs are not rank-ordered strictly according to STC values obtained in the T-maze, especially in the case of convulsants and antinicotinics, which are placed below hallucinogens and stimulants. The decision to order the drugs as shown is based on data obtained in bar-pressing tasks, which show hallucinogens and stimulants to be quite discriminable [18, 54]. In any case the rank-ordering should be regarded as approximate.

A list of published studies on the various drugs appears in Column 5 of Table 1. Many publications report data obtained with several different drugs. In order to avoid too many multiple entries, such publications are listed only in connection with the drugs about which they provide most information. Tasks other than the T-maze have yielded little data allowing a quantitative comparison of the discriminability of dissimilar drugs. They do, however, provide information about the degree to which the discriminable effects of various drugs are interchangeable or overlap.

A few comments may lend perspective on the Table. First, drugs do differ markedly in their discriminability despite the errors in precise rank-ordering which are undoubtedly present. The amount of SDL produced by drugs at the bottom of the Table appears to be at least an order of magnitude less than that produced by drugs near the top. Second, at least half the drugs in the Table are strongly discriminable. The published literature contains no reported failure to rapidly obtain drug-controlled responding when any drugs in the upper half of the Table are used in reasonable doses. Third, most of the drugs with readily discriminable effects are subject to abuse by man, and many have been self-administered by rats and monkeys. Conversely, most of the drugs with weakly discriminable effects are not subject to abuse and are not self-administered. This rather rough correlation is presently the only datum suggesting that SDL may be related to drug abuse.

It may be worthwhile to point out explicitly some exceptions to the overall correlation between discriminability and abuse. Antimuscarinics such as scopola-mine are quite discriminable, and have been shown to produce frank SDL amnesias. Nonetheless, they are seldom abused, perhaps because they produce a rather aversive high. Benzodiazepines are readily discriminable, but seldom abused by man. However, these drugs are self-administered by monkeys, and their low abuse potential in man may result from their slow onset of action. Finally, caffeine has weakly discriminable effects, although it could be classified as an abused drug. Considering the many factors which presumably influence drug abuse, these discrepancies do not seem to argue too strongly against the existence of an overall correlation between abuse and discriminability. The most alarming feature of the data is the fact that so many publications still leave us with a relatively weak data base for comparing the discriminability of different drugs.

Data on narcotics. Very few data are available on the discriminability of narcotics or on SDL produced by these drugs. An early study by Belleville showed a symmetrical SDL effect produced by morphine; in that study, rats were trained to bar-press for food on a VI schedule and then tested under extinction conditions with or without a change in drug condition [5]. More recently, Hill was unable to demonstrate a frank SDL amnesia using the shock escape T-maze task and morphine 4.5–36 mg/kg. However, he was able to establish drug discriminations with morphine, and discriminability was related to dose [20]. Differential responding did not develop as rapidly as with high doses of barbiturates, a finding replicated in this laboratory.

Despite the early report by Belleville, no other data have been published regarding the discriminable effects of narcotics. In part this can be attributed to legal restrictions, as most SDL experiments have been done in psychology departments not licensed to use narcotics.

Methodological problems. It is important to know whether discriminability and abuse potential are correlated. Although the data presented above are the best available today, they are not totally convincing. Fortunately, it is possible to suggest some improvements in methodology at this time, although not all problems can be solved. A further discussion of methodology can be found elsewhere [40].

The T-maze shock escape task has several good properties. Acquisition of drug discriminations in this task is a rather routine process which leads to a quantitative estimate (STC) of drug discriminability. Also, this task is relatively immune to behaviorally toxic drug effects, as shown by the fact that discriminability can be tested at doses high enough to disrupt performance in many other tasks. It is unfortunate, however, to use behavioral toxicity in the T-maze to select the dose at which discriminability is compared across drugs, as such comparisons are obtained at doses where behaviorally toxic drug effects introduce maximal error into the measurement. Moreover, the dose is determined by different factors for different drugs. Animals may be unable to perform because they die, or because they are too cognitively disorganized to learn the task even though they are still capable of running, or because they are anesthetized. Seemingly an improved comparison between drugs would be obtained if some explicit measure of behavioral toxicity was generated in another task, and discriminability was then compared using doses which produced equal behavioral toxicity in this other task, and which were low enough to produce minimal toxicity in the T-maze.

Claims have been made for the superiority of operant tasks because of their apparent sensitivity to lower doses of drug [26, 54]. In the T-maze, foot shock tends to disorganize responses, leading to occasional errors [26], and the T-maze may not be well adapted to measuring weak discriminable effects, at least when electric shock is used to motivate behavior. However, more prolonged training is required in other tasks, and the T-maze may be used to evaluate the discriminability of relatively low drug doses if training is similarly prolonged [38, 39]. More important, investigators using operant tasks have not yet developed their technique to the point where the rate of acquisition of a drug discrimination can yield a quantitative estimate of drug discriminability [4, 18, 27]. Quantitative measures derived from transfer tests administered to previously trained animals are possible, but are not useful for our present purposes [40].

In any case, the most important issue does not seem to be absolute sensitivity, but rather the ratio between the dose at which discriminability is easily studied and that at which behaviorally toxic effects disrupt task performance. In this respect, the T-maze task appears at least as good as other tasks presently in use, if not better.

Available data seriously raise the question whether all drug discrimination tasks will provide the same rank-ordering of drug discriminability when comparison is made across drugs. Studies using operant drug discrimination tasks suggest that amphetamine is more discriminable than pentobarbital, whereas the reverse is true in the T-maze. However, this may simply reflect the fact that depressant effects of pentobarbital produce relatively more behavioral toxicity in bar-pressing tasks than in the T-maze. It may be noted that the dose response curve for pentobarbital's discriminability has a steeper slope than that obtained with many other drugs, so that discriminability attenuates rapidly as dosage is reduced [38]. In any case, a serious effort to relate discriminability to abuse by comparison across drugs should apparently employ more than one drug discrimination task, because of the possibility of task differences.

A serious problem is raised by the lack of a generally accepted method for determining the relative abuse potential of different drugs. Such techniques are now being developed by investigators studying self-administration of drugs by animals [23]. However, a systematic rank-ordering of drugs according to their potency for self-administration has not yet been achieved. Hence, even if discriminability can be compared across drugs, the data regarding abuse are as yet inadequate to allow a rigorous test for a correlation between discriminability and abuse.

It may be possible to study the relationship between discriminability and abuse without resorting to comparisons between drugs. Specifically, if a manipulation can be found which varies the discriminability of a drug state, this can be tested to see if it also varies potency for self-administration. For example, the effects of various brain lesions on drug discriminability have been tested to see if a lesion could be found that would alter drug discriminability; so far this research has not met with success. It may be noted that the use of antagonists and blocking agents does not meet the requirements of this experimental strategy. While such agents do block the discriminable effects of drugs [30, 37, 50], they block many other drug effects as well. Rather than reducing the discriminability of a given dose of drug, their net effect is essentially to reduce the strength of drug action on the brain. What is needed is a manipulation which will alter discriminability without eliminating other drug effects. No such manipulations have been found.

REVIEW OF THEORIES

The mechanism producing SDL and drug discriminations is not known, and various theories have been put forward to explain these phenomena. Some of these theories are relevant to the apparent correlation between discriminability and abuse [17, 39]. It may be useful to briefly review the major hypotheses regarding the causes of SDL, with special emphasis on those that relate to abuse. It should be noted that these theories for the most part have not been testable, and the publications cited in connection with each theory are either the original sources of the theory or report data incompatible with it.

Theories Suggesting No Relationship

The phenomenon of SDL has been known since 1937 [15], and investigators attempting to rationalize its occurrence have proposed the following theories, which are essentially unrelated to drug abuse.

1. Drug-induced interoceptive stimuli produce SDL. The notion is that SDL and drug discriminations must reflect some variety of stimulus control, and that the relevant sensory stimuli enter the brain via the classic sensory pathways. Representative postulated internal stimuli include dry mouth, gastric contractions, vasodilation, etc. [32, 38].

2. Altered perception of environmental or of internal stimuli mediate SDL. According to this theory, drugs do not produce stimuli, but rather alter the perceptual processing of stimuli; e.g., by blurring vision or by making the rat analgesic [36, 38].

3. Areas of brain especially sensitive to drug become "drug receptors," and learning in other parts of the brain becomes conditional on their altered activity. For example, drug action on the reticular formation might produce massive changes in its efferent outflow to the cortex, and learned behaviors might be contingent on this abnormal cortical input. Such input need not be perceived as a sensation [33].

4. Drugs functionally ablate various structures normally involved in the learning process. Dissociated learning is accomplished by the remaining functional portions of the brain [6, 15, 38].

5. SDL occurs because drugs disrupt certain cognitive functions. The animal learns the required response by using the residual brain functions. However, the task is learned by some different strategy or encoding process than would normally be used if the brain were intact. In some sense, one may say that the drug changes the task by making the animal insensitive to certain aspects of it [43, 56].

6. The cell assemblies which mediate learned responses are state dependent because the synaptic changes which establish such cell assemblies are only appropriate to allow them to operate under the conditions of excitability present at the time of learning [32, 41].

7. Drug effects mimic naturally occurring internal states (e.g., arousal, hunger, thirst) which in turn acquire response control [14, 32, 38]. The notion

is that neural mechanisms allowing such states to control behavior exist, and that drugs use the same mechanisms to produce SDL.

Correlated but Not Causally Related

The apparent relationship between discriminability and abuse leads to the suggestion that both are caused by the same drug actions. This does not imply that SDL causes abuse or vice versa, but only that discriminability results from effects which are also reinforcing.

This notion has far-reaching implications if one accepts a hedonic theory for self-administration. If both SDL and drug abuse are produced by drug-induced hedonic affects, it may follow that recall should be "affect-specific," even if the affects are induced by manipulations other than drugs. However, except for a few studies on drive discriminations [31, 55] and some clinical observations in manic depressives [10], evidence of such affect-specific recall is strikingly absent. Nonetheless this extension of the theory has some virtue, as it is testable. Altered affective states can be induced by behavioral manipulations and by electrical stimulation of the brain.

Correlated and Indirectly Causal

Two theories have been put forward suggesting that discriminability may indirectly cause drug abuse [17, 39].

One theory proposes that an altered repertoire of drug-state responses develops with repeated drug use. If the drug-specific behaviors are more reinforcing than normal undrugged behaviors, then the subject may use drug to gain access to the drug response repertoire rather than because of any intrinsically reinforcing drug effects. This theory comes in two versions. The first postulates that a unique drug response repertoire is developed because environmental reinforcement contingencies are changed while the subject is drugged; e.g., because other people treat an intoxicated person differently than they treat an undrugged person. The second version proposes that drug alters the user's sensitivity to social reinforcement so that reinforcement contingencies are effectively changed even in the absence of any real change in the external environment. The theory provides a mechanism by which drugs initially possessing few reinforcing effects can become more reinforcing after prolonged use because of the desirability of behaviors linked to the drug condition.

Another theory which attributes a causal role in abuse to the stimulus properties of drugs regards the drug as a conditioned stimulus. For example, if early experience with an initially neutral drug is associated with positive social reinforcement, repeated drug experience may establish a conditioned association such that the drug becomes able to evoke the positive affect. This theory is somewhat tangential to our discussion of discriminative drug effects, as it treats the drug as a conditioned stimulus which evokes a reinforcing affect rather than as a discriminative stimulus. However, drugs can act as conditioned stimuli [13], and this may be related to their discriminable effects.

Correlated and Directly Causal

One final theory proposes that SDL is a directly causal factor in drug abuse. The notion is that the dissociative barrier prevents recall in the nondrug state for many of the negative consequences of drug use. Only the initial effects of the drug are well recalled—i.e., those which take place before a substantial change in state has occurred. Evidence supporting this proposal has been obtained by Tamerin et al., who showed that alcoholics selectively fail to remember much of the dysphoric content of their drinking episodes [53].

SUMMARY

Research on state-dependent learning and drug discriminations has progressed to the point where it is possible to make some tentative statements about the relative discriminability of various centrally acting drugs. The data suggest that the discriminability of various drugs is correlated with their potential for abuse. Some improvements in methodology are possible which may permit a more rigorous evaluation of this apparent correlation. Several theories seek to explain the apparent correlation between discriminability and abuse. Some of these theories suggest that state-dependent learning is one of the factors causing drug abuse.

REFERENCES

1. Barry, H. Prolonged measurements of discrimination between alcohol and nondrug states. *J. Comp. Physiol. Psychol.*, 65, 349–352, 1968.
2. Barry, H., Koepfer, E., & Lutch, J. Learning to discriminate between alcohol and nondrug condition. *Psychol. Rep.,* 16, 1072, 1965.
3. Barry, H., & Krimmer, E. C. Pentobarbital effects perceived by rats as resembling several other depressants but not alcohol. *Proc. 80th Amer. Psychol. Ass.,* 849–850, 1972.
4. Barry, H., & Kubena, R. K. Discriminative stimulus characteristics of alcohol, marihuana and atropine. In J. M. Singh, L. Miller, & H. Lal (Eds.), *Drug addiction.* Vol. 1. *Experimental pharmacology.* Mt. Kisco, N. Y.: Futura Pub. Co., 1972.
5. Belleville, R. E. Control of behavior by drug-produced internal stimuli. *Psychopharmacologia,* 5, 95–105, 1964.
6. Berger, B., & Stein, L. Asymmetrical dissociation of learning between scopolamine and Wy 4036, a new benzodiazepine tranquilizer. *Psychopharmacologia* (Berl.), 14, 351–358, 1969.
7. Bliss, D. K., Sledjeski, M., & Leiman, A. State dependent choice behavior in the rhesus monkey. *Neuropsychologica,* 9, 51–59, 1971.
8. Brown, A., Feldman, R. S., & Moore, J. W. Conditional discrimination learning based upon chlordiazepoxide: Dissociation or cue? *J. Comp. Physiol. Psychol.,* 66, 211–215, 1968.
9. Bueno, O. F. A., and Carlini, E. A. Dissociation of learning in marihuana tolerant rats. *Psychopharmacologia* (Berl.), 25, 49–56, 1972.
10. Bunney, W. E., Jr., & Hartmann, E. L. Study of a patient with 48-hour manic depressive cycles: 1. An analysis of behavioral factors. *Arch. Gen. Psychiat.,* 12, 611–618, 1965.

11. Cherkashin, A. N., & Azarasvili, A. A. Dissociated learning in animals. *Soviet Psychology*, **10**, 303–314, 1972.
12. Conger, J. The effects of alcohol on conflict behavior in the albino rat. *Quart. J. Stud. Alcohol*, **12**, 1–29, 1951.
13. Cook, L., Davidson, A., Davis, D. J., & Kelleher, R. T. Epinephrine, norepinephrine, and acetylcholine as conditioned stimuli for avoidance behavior. *Science*, **131**, 990–992, 1960.
14. Fischer, R., & Landon, G. M. On the arousal state-dependent recall of "subconscious" experience: stateboundness. *British J. Psychiatry*, **120**, 159–172, 1972.
15. Girden, E., & Culler, E. A. Conditioned responses in curarized striate muscle in dogs. *J. Comp. Psychol.*, **23**, 261–274, 1937.
16. Harris, R. T., & Balster, R. L. Discriminative control by *dl*-amphetamine and saline of lever choice and response patterning. *Psychon. Sci.*, **10**, 105–106, 1968.
17. Harris, R. T., & Balster, R. L. An analysis of psychological dependence. In R. T. Harris, W. N. McIsaac, & C. R. Schuster, Jr. (Eds.), *Advances in mental science II: Drug dependence*. Austin: University of Texas Press, 1970.
18. Harris, R. T., & Balster, R. L. An analysis of the function of drugs in the stimulus control of operant behavior. In T. Thompson & R. Pickens (Eds.), *Stimulus properties of drugs*. New York: Appleton-Century-Crofts, 1971.
19. Henriksson, B. J., & Jarbe, T. Delta⁹-tetrahydrocannabinol used as discriminative stimulus for rats in position learning in a T-shaped water maze. *Psychon. Sci.*, **27**, 25–26, 1972.
20. Hill, H. E., Jones, B. E., & Bell, E. C. State-dependent control of discrimination by morphine and pentobarbital. *Psychopharmacologia*, **22**, 305–313, 1971.
21. Hirschhorn, I. D., & Winter, J. C. Mescaline and lysergic acid diethylamide (LSD) as discriminative stimuli. *Psychopharmacologia* (Berl.), **22**, 64–71, 1971.
22. Hurst, P. M., Radlow, R., Chubb, N. C., & Bagley, S. K. Effects of *d*-amphetamine on acquisition, persistence and recall. *Am. J. Psychol.*, **82**, 307–319, 1969.
23. Johanson, C. E. Choice of cocaine by rhesus monkeys as a function of dosage. *Proceedings of 79th Amer. Psychol. Ass.*, 751–752, 1971.
24. John, E. R. State-dependent learning. In *Mechanisms of memory*. New York: Academic Press, 1967.
25. Kilbey, M. Marlyne, Harris, R. T., & Aigner, T. G. Establishment of equivalent external and internal stimulus control of an operant behavior and its reversal. *Proceedings of 79th Amer. Psychol. Ass.*, 767–768, 1971.
26. Kubena, R. K., & Barry, H. Generalization by rats of alcohol and atropine stimulus characteristics to other drugs. *Psychopharmacologia*, **15**, 196–206, 1969.
27. Kubena, R. K., & Barry, H. Two procedures for training differential responses in alcohol and nondrug conditions. *J. Pharm. Sci.*, **58**, 99–101, 1969.
28. Kubena, R. K., & Barry, H. Stimulus characteristics of marihuana components. *Nature*, **235**, 397–398, 1972.
29. Ley, P., Jain, V. K., Swinson, R. P., Eaves, D., Bradshaw, P. W., Kincey, J. A., Crowder, R., & Abbiss, S. A state-dependent learning effect produced by amylobarbitone sodium. *Brit. J. Psychiat.*, **120**, 511–515, 1972.
30. Morrison, C. F., & Stephenson, J. A. Nicotine injections as the conditioned stimulus in discrimination learning. *Psychopharmologia* (Berl.), **15**, 351–360, 1969.
31. Otis, L. S. Drive conditioning: Fear as a response to biogenic drive stimuli previously associated with painful stimulation. *Amer. Psychol.*, **11**, 397, 1956. (Abstract)
32. Overton, D. A. State-dependent or "dissociated" learning produced with pentobarbital. *J. Comp. Physiol. Psychol.*, **57**, 3–12, 1964.
33. Overton, D. A. State-dependent learning produced by depressant and atropine-like drugs. *Psychopharmacologia* (Berl.), **10**, 6–31, 1966.

34. Overton, D. A. Differential responding in a three choice maze controlled by three drug states. *Psychopharmacologia* (Berl.), **11**, 376–378, 1967.
35. Overton, D. A. Dissociated learning in drug states (state-dependent learning). In D. H. Efron, J. O. Cole, J. Levine, & R. Wittenborn (Eds.), *Psychopharmacology, A review of progress, 1957–1967.* (USPHS Pub. No. 1836) Washington, D.C.: U.S. Government Printing Office, 1968.
36. Overton, D. A. Visual cues and shock sensitivity in the control of T-maze choice by drug conditions. *J. Comp. Physiol. Psychol.*, **66**, 216–219, 1968.
37. Overton, D. A. Control of T-maze choice by nicotinic, antinicotinic, and antimuscarinic drugs. *Proceedings of the 77th Annual Convention of the Amer. Psychol. Ass.*, 869–870, 1969.
38. Overton, D. A. Discriminative control of behavior by drug states. In T. Thompson & R. Pickens (Eds.), *Stimulus properties of drugs.* New York: Appleton-Century-Crofts, 1971.
39. Overton, D. A. State dependent learning produced by alcohol and its relevance to alcoholism. In B. Kissen & H. Begleiter (Eds.), *The biology of alcoholism.* Vol. 2. *Physiology and behavior.* New York: Plenum Press, 1972.
40. Overton, D. A. Experimental methods for the study of state dependent learning. *Federation Proceedings*, 1974, submitted.
41. Pusakulich, R. L., & Nielson, H. C. Neural thresholds and state-dependent learning. *Exper. Neurol.*, **34**, 33–44, 1972.
42. Reichert, H. Evidence for a memory consolidation interpretation of state dependent learning. *Dissertation Abstracts Internat.*, **32**(2-B), 1255, 1971.
43. Sachs, E. Dissociation of learning in rats and its similarities to dissociative states in man. In J. Zubin & H. Hunt (Eds.), *Comparative Psychopathology.* New York: Grune & Stratton, 1967.
44. Schechter, M. D., & Rosecrans, J. A. Behavioral evidence for two types of cholinergic receptors in the CNS. *Europ. J. Pharm.*, **15**, 375–378, 1971.
45. Schechter, M. D., & Rosecrans, J. A. CNS effect of nicotine as the discriminative stimulus for the rat in a T-maze. *Life Sci.*, **10**, 821–832, 1971.
46. Schechter, M. D., & Rosecrans, J. A. Atropine antagonism of arecoline-cued behavior in the rat. *Life Sci.*, **11**, 517–523, 1972.
47. Schechter, M. D., & Rosecrans, J, A. Effect of mecamylamine on discrimination between nicotine-and arecoline-produced cues. *Europ. J. Pharm.*, **17**, 179–182, 1972.
48. Schechter, M. D., & Rosecrans, J. A. Lysergic acid diethylamide (LSD) as a discriminative cue: drugs with similar stimulus properties. *Psychopharmacologia* (Berl.), **26**, 313–316, 1972.
49. Schechter, M. D., & Rosecrans, J. A. Nicotine as a discriminative cue in rats: Inability of related drugs to produce a nicotine-like cueing effect. *Psychopharmacologia* (Berl.), **27**, 379–387, 1972.
50. Schechter, M. D., & Rosecrans, J. A. Nicotine as a discriminative stimulus in rats depleted of norepinephrine or 5-hydroxytryptamine. *Psychopharmacologia* (Berl.), **24**, 417–429, 1972.
51. Stewart, Jane. Differential responses based on the physiological consequences of pharmacological agents. *Psychopharmacologia*, **3**, 132–138, 1962.
52. Stewart, Jane, Krebs, W. H., & Kaczender, Elizabeth. State-dependent learning produced with steroids. *Nature*, **216**, 1223–1224, 1967.
53. Tamerin, J. S., Weiner, S., Poppen, R., Steinglass, P., & Mendelson, J. H. Alcohol and memory: Amnesia and short-term memory function during experimentally induced intoxication. *Amer. J. Psychiat.*, **127**, 1659–1664, 1971.
54. Waters, W. H., Richards, D. W. III, and Harris, R. T. Discriminative control and generalization of the stimulus properties of D,L-amphetamine in the rat. In J. M. Singh, L. Miller, & H. Lal (Eds.), *Drug addiction.* Vol. 1. *Experimental pharmacology.* Mt. Kisco, N. Y.: Futura Pub. Co., 1972.

55. Webb, W. B. Drive stimuli as cues. *Psychol. Rep.,* 1, 287–298, 1955.
56. Weingartner, H., & Faillace, L. A. Alcohol state-dependent learning in man. *J. Ner. Ment. Dis.,* 153, 395–406, 1971.
57. White, R. P., Nash, C. B., Westerbeke, E. J., & Possanza, G. J. Phylogenetic comparison of central actions produced by different doses of atropine and hyoscine. *Arch. Int. Pharmacodyn.,* 132, 349–363, 1961.

BEHAVIORAL ANALYSIS OF OPIATE DEPENDENCE[1]

Charles R. Schuster and Chris E. Johanson
University of Chicago

At the 1967 American College of Neuropsychopharmacology meetings a review of "The Experimental Analysis of Opioid Dependence" was presented and published in the volume *Psychopharmacology: A Review of Progress, 1957-1967* [41]. The subsequent five-year period has increasingly affirmed our conviction that the behavioral aspects of drug abuse can best be analyzed within the conceptual framework of behavioral analyses utilizing the principles of both operant and classical conditioning [37]. The fundamental principle underlying operant conditioning is that certain aspects of behavior are controlled by their consequences. Behavior controlled by its consequences is termed operant behavior, and the controlling consequence for the operant behavior is defined as a reinforcer. Within this framework drugs are viewed as reinforcers capable of controlling behavior in the same manner as conventional reinforcers (food, water, etc.). One of the major advantages of such an analysis is that it enables the experimenter to utilize a wide range of data derived from the analysis of behavior maintained by these other reinforcers.

Classical conditioning involves the pairing of a stimulus (unconditioned), which elicits some unconditioned behavioral response, with a neutral stimulus. After repeated pairing of these two stimulus events, the neutral stimulus presented alone may elicit the behavioral response. In such a case, the neutral stimulus is termed a conditioned stimulus and the behavior is considered classically conditioned. A variety of responses to drugs can be classically conditioned

[1] Supported by USPHS grants MH-18,245 and MH-11,042 awarded to Charles R. Schuster, Ph.D., and MH-22,971 awarded to the Department of Psychiatry, University of Chicago (Daniel X. Freedman, Principal Investigator).

and a full understanding of the phenomenon of drug abuse must take this into account. Such classical conditioning is relevant in the present context to the extent that it may influence the reinforcing actions of a drug.

The principal goal of the experimental analysis of the behavioral aspects of drug abuse is the determination of biological and environmental variables which modify a drug's reinforcing efficacy, that is, the extent to which a drug is self-administered. It is our purpose here to review selectively those variables affecting the acquisition and maintenance of opiate self-administration behavior. Studies of general pharmacology and neurochemistry will be discussed only where they enable us to illustrate a behavioral principle.

Table 1 presents a summary of the classes of variables which have been shown to affect operant behavior in general, and drug self-administration in particular. It is our intention to review the literature on the behavioral aspects of opiate dependence using this conceptual framework.

I. Reinforcement Variables

A. *Delay of reinforcement.* There have been no direct investigations of the acquisition and maintenance of a drug-reinforced operant response when a delay is introduced between the response and the delivery of the drug reinforcement. However, investigation of other reinforcers has shown that the delay of reinforcement is a significant variable; both acquisition and maintenance of behavior are weakened as a function of delay of reinforcement [43]. It seems likely that this variable would have a similar effect when drugs are used as

TABLE 1

Principal Variables Affecting Drug Self-Administration

| I. Reinforcement Variables
  A. Delay of reinforcement
  B. Magnitude of reinforcement
  C. Rate of delivery

II. Antecedent Conditions
  A. Deprivation
  B. Satiation

III. Organismic Variables
  A. Genotype
  B. Species
  C. Age
  D. Sex | IV. Current Environmental
  Contingency Variables
  A. Schedule of positive
    reinforcement
  B. Extinction
  C. Punishment

V. Experiential Variables
  A. Pharmacological
    1. Tolerance
    2. Physical dependence and
      withdrawal
    3. Prior self-administration
  B. Behavioral
    1. Conditioned withdrawal
    2. Conditioned opiate effects |

reinforcers. From a theoretical viewpoint this variable may account for the ease of conditioning animals to lever-press for opiate reinforcement delivered intravenously relative to giving the drug orally [40]. From a practical viewpoint, it would appear that a drug which could not be taken intravenously and which had a slow onset of action after oral ingestion should have a low abuse potential—a contention partly substantiated by the finding that barbiturates with faster onset of action are preferred by barbiturate abusers [23]. Given the technology of pharmaceutical chemistry, it should not be difficult to modify currently abused drugs as well as to develop new ones with these characteristics. However, the behavior analysis literature has also shown that behavior can be maintained, even with a 24-hour delay, if conditions are suitably arranged [2, 12]. It remains to be seen, however, whether behavior can initially be acquired with such delays.

   B. *Magnitude of reinforcement.* Magnitude of reinforcement has been most systematically investigated in procedures where the drug is infused through an indwelling venous catheter. The relationship between rate of responding and magnitude of drug reinforcement varies with different classes of drugs [37, 47]. Weeks [48], Weeks and Collins [49], and Collins and Weeks [8] reported that the response rate of rats reinforced with morphine on a fixed-ratio schedule was inversely related to dose in the range of 3.2 to 10.0 mg/kg-infusion. Woods and Schuster [50], using rhesus monkeys, found that rate of responding for morphine delivered on a variable-interval schedule showed an inverted U-shaped function when dosage was varied across a range from 10 to 1000 ug/kg-infusion. It is important to note that the rhesus monkeys in this study were physically dependent upon and tolerant to morphine at doses above 10 ug/kg-infusion. Clearly, tolerance development to the depressant actions of morphine could alter the slope of the function relating response rate to the magnitude (unit dose) of morphine reinforcement. In a more recent study using monkeys not physically dependent and only minimally tolerant, Balster, Schuster, and Wilson [5] also showed an inverse function relating fixed-ratio response rate to the magnitude of morphine, propoxyphene, and codeine reinforcement. A direct comparison of these two studies is not possible due to differences in procedure and dose range tested. However, it appears that the function relating response rate and unit dose is shifted to the left for nontolerant monkeys. In addition, other observations (Schuster, 1968) indicate that the inverse portion of the function is steeper for nontolerant monkeys.

   C. *Rate of delivery of drug reinforcement.* There have been only two studies in which the rate of infusion of drug reinforcement has been investigated, and in neither study was an opiate used. Pickens and Thompson [33] varied the rate of infusion of methamphetamine in rats lever-pressing on a fixed-ratio schedule for intravenous drug reinforcement. They found that response rate was independent of rate of infusion over a range of 25 to 75 seconds. Balster and Schuster [4], however, using a more sensitive schedule of reinforcement (a fixed-interval schedule) with rhesus monkeys responding for intravenous cocaine found a direct function relating response rate and rate of infusion over a range of 5 to 200 seconds. Although the explanation of these findings is speculative, this variable should be investigated, with an opiate as the reinforcer. Such a study might indicate whether it is the onset effect (e.g., the "rush") or the more long-lasting action of the opiates (e.g., decreased food motivation) which is primarily reinforcing.

II. Antecedent Variables

A. *Deprivation.* The reinforcing efficacy of food, water, and sex has been demonstrated to be directly related to deprivation in various animal species. Similarly, deprivation of opiates in physically dependent animals markedly increases the reinforcing efficacy of morphine. Thompson and Schuster [46] found that increasing the deprivation of rhesus monkeys from 6 to 24 hours produced a marked increase in the rate of responding on a fixed-interval, fixed-ratio chained schedule of morphine reinforcement. Opiate deprivation can also be produced by the administration of opiate antagonists. In the same study, Thompson and Schuster found that comparable increases in rate were obtained by morphine deprivation and nalorphine pretreatment. In addition, Weeks [48] and Weeks and Collins [49] reported that administration of nalorphine to rats self-administering morphine produced increases in response rate on a ratio schedule comparable with that observed following morphine deprivation. Goldberg, Woods, and Schuster [19] reported that this action of nalorphine was dose-dependent. At low doses (30–300 ug/kg) nalorphine caused an increase in morphine-reinforced lever-pressing by physically dependent rhesus monkeys. At higher doses, however, the animals showed a dose-related depression in responding for morphine reinforcement under limited access conditions. These findings will be discussed in greater detail in relationship to procedures for weakening self-administration behavior.

B. *Satiation.* In addition to drug deprivation used to control motivational conditions, animals may be pretreated (e.g., satiated) with graded amounts of the agent used as the reinforcer. Thompson and Schuster [46] pretreated physically dependent monkeys with 2, 4, or 6 mg/kg of morphine 45 minutes before the periods when the animals were scheduled to self-administer morphine. They found that the length of time required to complete the morphine-reinforced fixed-ratio 25 varied directly with the pretreatment dosage. Thompson [45] also found that hourly intramuscular injections of the opioid, methadone, suppressed morphine-reinforced responding by monkeys. Weeks and Collins [49] have reported that etonitazine introduced into drinking water, or continuously infused intravenously, suppressed morphine-reinforced lever-pressing by physically dependent rats. In addition, continuous infusions of codeine and meperidine also suppressed morphine self-administration. Dex-oxadrol, a clinically effective nonopioid analgesic, was found ineffective in suppressing morphine self-administration, as was the opioid, dextromethorphan, which has minimal abuse liability in humans [9].

Thus, satiating the organism with drug decreases the probability that the organism will seek further drug reinforcement. This is, of course, one of the mechanisms underlying the clinical efficacy of methadone in the treatment of heroin dependence.

III. Organismic Variables

A. *Genotype.* While obviously all humans can be *made* physically dependent upon opiates, the propensity of the individual to seek out the opiate and to self-administer it varies markedly from one person to another. Whether such differences are in any way influenced by genetic factors is at this point unknown. Nichols and Hsiao [32] report that rats can be selectively bred for their ability to be conditioned to drink a morphine solution. Inbreeding of "susceptible" rats produced animals with an increasing tendency to drink morphine over successive generations. Further, inbreeding of "resistant" animals produced a strain of animals showing a very low probability of morphine ingestion. Nichols and Hsiao, in addition, reported that "susceptible" animals in the F-3 generation would drink significantly greater amounts of alcohol than animals from the strain "resistant" to morphine. Further studies ruled out the influence of differences in emotionality or maternal care. However, Nichols [31] also reported that "susceptible" rats make fewer errors than "non-susceptible" animals in learning maze problems. It seems possible, therefore, that differences in the ability to learn to ingest morphine could be related to the ability to bridge the temporal delay between the drinking response and the pharmacological actions of morphine responsible for reinforcement. It would be important to determine whether the strain differences in rats would hold up if the drug reinforcement were delivered intravenously where delay of reinforcement is minimal and learning may be easier.

B. *Species.* Most studies of intravenous opiate self-administration have used either rats or rhesus monkeys as the subjects. By and large these two species behave similarly in terms of self-administration, except that for rats the intake is higher, and higher doses per infusion can be tolerated. In a recent paper, Jones and Prada [25] reported that a large percentage of dogs tested will not self-administer morphine when it is available via an intravenous catheter. In this regard they differ from rhesus monkeys and rats, since the vast majority of the latter species will lever-press for morphine reinforcement without any prior experience with the drug [11, 48, 50]. Jones and Prada did find, however, that dogs who learned to lever-press for morphine, after having been made physically dependent by the experimenter, would "relapse" to morphine self-administration 1 to 6 months later. They contend, therefore, that the dog is an excellent subject for studying "relapse" to opiate self-administration following a period of enforced abstinence. This contention seems bas d on the notion that only a small percentage of humans exposed to opiates will abuse them unless social conditions "force" them to do so. These pressures are comparable to the experimenter administering morphine to the dogs noncontingently. If humans, like dogs, do become addicted in a nonvoluntary way, they will invariably relapse following a period of enforced abstinence. Unfortunately, the question of which animals—monkeys, rats, or dogs—are the best models for the study of drug abuse is unanswerable until there is a better description of the human problem and a more careful simulation of all the consequences of illicit drug taking.

C. Age. Only one study has been conducted to determine whether age is a variable affecting opiate self-administration. Nichols [30] reported that rats conditioned to drink morphine showed a decline in intake with increasing age. The significance of this finding awaits a more precise specification of the correlated physiological changes which occur with age.

D. Sex. Up to this time, there have been no systematic studies of opiate self-administration in animals of different sex. The clinical observation of a markedly greater incidence of heroin addiction in males could be due either to differences in endocrine functioning or to differences in their social roles. Clearly, the use of animal subjects would enable these factors to be experimentally separated.

IV. Current Environmental Contingencies

A. Schedule of reinforcement. The frequency of occurrence and specific patterning of behavior and its persistence are to a large extent a function of the existing schedule of reinforcement [13, 43]. Although most studies designed to elucidate the variables controlling behavior have used conventional reinforcers, one would expect these relations to hold when opiates are used as reinforcers. Drugs, however, have some unique properties in that they have a number of behavioral effects in addition to acting as reinforcers. These other effects may very well include effects upon the rate of emission of the response producing drug reinforcement. An extreme example of this would be a situation in which the drug reinforcement was at a high enough dosage to produce unconsciousness. The duration of the drug-induced unconsciousness would of course be the most potent variable determining the rate and pattern of emission of the drug-reinforced response. Drugs at lower dosages may have more subtle but nonetheless potent effects upon the patterning and rate of emission of the drug self-administration behavior. This is undoubtedly the case with opiates. For instance, opiates generally depress an organism's rate of emission of operant responding for food [51] in a dose-dependent manner. Similarly, rate of responding for opiate reinforcement is an inverse function of dose per reinforcement [5, 51]. The lower response rate for higher dosages of opiates, therefore, does not seem to indicate less reinforcing efficacy; rather, it is an indication of the direct suppressant effect of opiates, the duration and intensity of which increase as a function of dosage. This suppressant effect is a potent determinant of rate of responding regardless of the nature of the reinforcer. The situation is further complicated in the case of opiates by the development of tolerance or physical dependence. As discussed earlier, these factors can alter the shape of the function relating dosage of opiate reinforcement to response rate. As a result, we cannot assess reinforcing efficacy using rate as a measure, particularly when attempting to compare different drugs.

In order to bypass the problems of using rate as a measure of reinforcing efficacy, several investigators are now developing preference procedures [3, 14, 24]. Although the details of these three procedures differ greatly, two aspects are important: (a) the organism is given a simultaneous paired choice between different drug solutions, and (b) the organism is offered this choice at a time when he is *relatively* free of the rate-modifying effects of a drug. Use of these preference procedures has shown that higher dosages of psychomotor-stimulant drugs are chosen over low dosages [24]. This finding is in contrast to the inverse relationship of response rate to magnitude of reinforcement (dosage). To date, these choice procedures have not been used to determine the comparative reinforcing efficacy of various opiates. Clearly, this is an area that needs investigation.

Despite the problems of using rate of responding as a dependent variable for drug reinforcement, various schedules of reinforcement have been investigated. In the main, the patterns of responding generated by ratio schedules for morphine, methadone, and codeine [51] are similar to those seen for food reinforcement. Woods and Schuster [50] used a variable-interval schedule of morphine reinforcement to study the effects of dosage in the rhesus monkey. This schedule generated a pattern of responding characteristic of interval schedules, but rate at all dosages of morphine was markedly below that generated by food reinforcement on the same variable-interval schedule in the same animals. Again, this is probably a reflection of the rate-suppressant effects of an opiate reinforcer.

Two studies have been reported involving more complex schedules. Thompson and Schuster [46] used a fixed-interval, fixed-ratio chained schedule of intravenous morphine reinforcement with monkeys. The behavior was characteristic of that generated by chained schedules and commonly observed with use of other reinforcers. Recent investigations of highly complex multioperant sequences in which morphine is the terminal reinforcer have been described by Thompson and Pickens [45a]. In this case monkeys performed a chain of heterogeneous responses beginning with standing on a platform scale, followed by opening and closing a door to a compartment, cooperating with another monkey in holding a switch closed, and finally, operating a lever on a fixed-ratio schedule for intravenous morphine. This behavior is well maintained, with pausing during the early components varying with the terminal ratio requirement.

   B. *Extinction.* One of the principal means of decreasing the frequency of occurrence of an operant is to sever its temporal connection with the reinforcer maintaining it. In the case of opiate reinforcement this can be accomplished in two ways: (a) by substituting an inert substance such as saline for the drug, or (b) by pretreating the organism with another drug (e.g., an opiate antagonist) which prevents the opiate from exerting its reinforcing effect.

Woods and Schuster [51] studied rate of responding in extinction following various dosages of morpine delivered on a variable-interval schedule of reinforcement. To extinguish the behavior, saline was substituted for the morphine solution, but in all other ways the schedule was unchanged. The number of responses in the first 3 days of extinction was a direct function of the dosage of morphine previously used as the reinforcer. In addition, at the lowest dosages (10 and 25 ug/kg-infusion) there were no signs that the animals had become physically dependent upon morphine. At the higher dosages (100, 250, 500, and 1,000 ug/kg-infusion) the animals showed definite signs of physical dependence, the intensity of which was a function of dose. Thus the increased response rate in extinction following the higher dosages of morphine reinforcement was probably a reflection of the dose-dependent physical "need" for the drug.

A second means of extinguishing an opiate-reinforced response is by pretreating the organism with a drug which prevents the opiate from exerting its reinforcing effect. It has been suggested that cyclazocine, an opiate antagonist, could be utilized clinically in the treatment of opiate dependence in this manner [28]. As yet, however, treatment procedures utilizing cyclazocine have had only limited success in the treatment of opiate dependence [15]. In principle, however, opiate antagonists represent an effective means of producing extinction of a response maintained by opiate reinforcement. In a study by Goldberg, Woods, and Schuster [19], monkeys self-administering morphine were chronically treated with various doses of nalorphine. At low dosages of nalorphine animals self-administered increased quantities of morphine. At higher doses the animals showed a typical extinction curve so that by the fifth day their intake of morphine approached zero. Unlike clinical patients receiving opiate antagonists, the animals in this study had no choice but to receive the antagonist. Clinically, however, this is not the case, since patients may choose not to return to the clinic for their medication.

Recently, Davis and Smith [10] reported the effects of pretreatment with alpha-methylparatyrosine (AMPT) in rats self-administering either amphetamine or morphine. Animals pretreated with AMPT failed to lever-press either for morphine or for amphetamine. Whether this effect of AMPT is a specific blocking of the reinforcing effects of morphine and amphetamine cannot be determined from this study. These investigators, however, interpret their data as an instance of extinction of the self-administration response.

C. *Punishment.* The most traditional means of handling the problem of illicit drug self-administration has been to suppress its occurrence through punishment. Our whole elaborate legal system of monetary fines and imprisonment (time out from certain positive reinforcers) is predicated on the efficacy of punishment as a means of controlling operant behavior. Unfortunately, there have been no systematic laboratory studies of the effects of punishment on opiate self-administration. However, we believe that certain extrapolations can be made from the classic studies of Azrin and his colleagues [1] who studied the effects of punishment on a food-reinforced operant. Briefly, these studies showed that operant behavior could be suppressed by electric-shock punishment if it occurred immediately following the response and if the intensity of the shock was high enough. Lower shock intensities produced a temporary suppression, but with continued experience the animals adapted to the punishment. If an alternative response which was not punished but produced the same reinforcer was allowed, then punishment at very low shock-intensity levels was effective. We are currently attempting to replicate these studies using both amphetamines and opiates as the reinforcer for the lever-pressing of rhesus monkeys. If these same functional relations hold for drugs as reinforcers we may be able to devise a more rational use of punishment as a means of controlling illicit drug self-administration.

V. Experiential Variables

Many actions of pharmacological agents are modified by past experiences of the organism. These experiential variables may be primarily pharmacological or behavioral; but they may be, as well, a complex interaction of the two.

A. *Pharmacological.* (1) Tolerance: Clearly an organism's self-administration of an opiate will be affected by the development of tolerance. Rhesus monkeys, allowed to self-administer morphine intravenously on a fixed-ratio schedule, show a gradual increase in total daily intake over the course of 4 to 6 weeks. Thereafter, intake of the drug remains stable [11]. This gradual increase in opiate intake over time has been reported, as well, for monkeys [6] and rats [27] ingesting morphine orally. These results are most likely a function of the development of tolerance to the depressant effects of morphine which initially limit the organism's ability to self-administer the drug. Schuster [36] and Woods and Schuster [51] have shown that in monkeys the number of days for reaching asymptotic responding for morphine reinforcement is a direct function of dosage per infusion. Thus at very low dosages (10 ug/kg-infusion) animals reach asymptotic responding within 3 days, whereas with dosages of 1000 ug/kg-infusion it may be 30 to 45 days before response rate is maximal. Studies of residual tolerance after drug-free periods have not been systematically conducted in relation to self-administration behavior. It seems likely, however, that some degree of tolerance should remain, and further that it would redevelop rapidly in a previously tolerant animal. As reported elsewhere in this book, tolerance following single injections of opiates has been observed for periods up to 15 months (see the Cochin chapter).

(2) Physical dependence: Temporally correlated with the development of tolerance to opiates is the development of physical dependence. It is beyond the scope of this review to discuss whether these two phenomena are mechanistically related. Our concern in this context is the influence of physical dependence on the self-administration of opiates. There are essentially two aspects to this

problem: (*a*) Is physical dependence a necessary antecedent condition for opiates to act as a reinforcer? (*b*) Does physical dependence influence the reinforcing efficacy of opiates? These questions have been extensively discussed elsewhere [36, 37, 40, 41, 51], and only the conclusions will be reviewed. It would appear that for rats and monkeys physical dependence is neither a necessary nor a sufficient condition for opiates to act as reinforcers. However, the reinforcing efficacy of opiates is markedly increased when physical dependence does develop. It seems that opiate self-administration in the physically dependent organism is reinforcing, first, because of the positively reinforcing pharmacological actions of morphine and, secondly, because of the ability of the drug to terminate the aversive aspects of withdrawal. Both these sources of reinforcement must be considered in analyzing self-administration behavior.

Opiate physical dependence has also been shown to determine whether certain other drugs will act as reinforcers. Many of the recently synthesized "opioids" have mixed agonist and antagonist actions. Pentazocine, shown to be a weak opiate antagonist, is also found to share many of the agonistic actions of opiates. Recently, Goldberg, Hoffmeister, and Schlichting [20] have shown that pentazocine acts as a positive reinforcer (i.e., will be self-administered) in nonphysically dependent rhesus monkeys. In animals physically dependent upon morphine, however, the drug acts as a negative reinforcer (i.e., animals lever-press to avoid an infusion of pentazocine). Thus, prior opiate physical dependence determined whether pentazocine would act as a positive or negative reinforcer in the rhesus monkey. This finding calls into question the interpretation of previous findings by Schuster et al. [38] who reported a low "abuse potential" for pentazocine in heroin-dependent street addicts.

(3) Prior self-administration of other drugs: Very often, in the laboratory (because of cost and efficiency) and on the "street" (because of availability), organisms self-administer a wide variety of drugs both in succession and in combination. To date, there have been no systematic studies of the self-administration of combinations of drugs. Recently, however, Schlichting, Goldberg, Wuttke, and Hoffmeister [35] have shown that different drug class histories have an effect on subsequent self-administration of amphetamine. All monkeys, regardless of their prior drug history, self-administered amphetamine; however, animals with a history of cocaine self-administration responded at higher rates for the higher dose of amphetamine (0.05 mg/kg) and tended to extinguish at the lowest dose (0.005 mg/kg) compared to monkeys with a history of codeine or pentobarbital self-administration. Patterns of amphetamine self-administration tended to be similar to the pattern of the previous drug; that is, the cocaine group took amphetamine at regular intervals, whereas the other two groups had both long and short inter-response times (i.e., irregular patterns). Hoffmeister and Schlichting [21] substituted several opiates (morphine and codeine) and opioids (pentazocine, propirom-fumarate, *d*-propoxyphene and nalorphine) in monkeys trained with either codeine or cocaine as the reinforcing

drug. At doses of the substituted drugs self-administered above saline rates, the codeine group self-administered more of each of the drugs than the cocaine group; the only exception was nalorphine, which neither group self-administered. In addition, lower doses of the drug tested were found to be reinforcers in the codeine group than in the cocaine group. The variables responsible for these differences are not known, but the data do indicate the importance of prior drug self-administration.

B. *Behavioral.* (1) Conditioned withdrawal: The role of conditioned withdrawal in the phenomenon of opiate dependence has been discussed extensively in this book (see the Wikler chapter). We will selectively review data to further illustrate the importance of this variable.

In 1952 Irwin and Seevers [22] reported that in monkeys dependent on methadone, ketobemidone, or racemorphan, which had repeatedly experienced nalorphine-induced withdrawal, an injection of saline elicited the withdrawal syndrome even after an opiate-free period of 1 to 2 months. They interpreted these results as indicating that through classical conditioning, the injection procedure (the CS) had acquired the ability to elicit the withdrawal response because of its temporal.association with nalorphine (the UCS).

Goldberg and Schuster [16] provided a further demonstration that at least certain aspects of the morphine withdrawal syndrome could be classically conditioned. Nalorphine (a UCS), when given to morphine-dependent monkeys working for food on an FR-10 schedule of reinforcement, caused a disruption in behavior. When a tone (the CS) was repeatedly presented 5 minutes before and after such an injection, it alone became capable of suppressing food-reinforced behavior. In addition, when saline injections were substituted for nalorphine, suppression during the tone persisted as long as 40 days. Bradycardia, emesis, and salivation were also conditioned by this procedure. This study demonstrates that stimuli in an addict's environment can elicit reactions similar to those elicited by withdrawal. Goldberg et al. [18] increased the generality of this finding by showing that the list of conditionable reactions included increased self-administration of morphine. Injections of certain dosages of nalorphine in morphine-dependent monkeys increase their rate of self-administration of morphine. When a flashing red light (CS) was paired with the nalorphine injections, eventually injections of saline accompanied by the light also resulted in increased morphine self-administration.

These studies are relevant for explaining some of the variables which contribute to the continual use of opiates in dependent persons; however, they say little about the relevance of conditioning in relapse. Goldberg and Schuster [17] have extended their work successfully in this area, using the same paradigm as in their original study [16]. They again found that a neutral stimulus, this time a red light, when paired with nalorphine injections, could produce, when presented alone, suppression of food-reinforced behavior. Next they discontinued morphine injections for 30 days and allowed animals to undergo withdrawal. When they returned the animals to the experimental situation, the red light alone suppressed food-responding; the effect persisted for 60 to 120 days and when finally extinguished was rapidly reconditioned. However, one important part of this study remains to be done. In order to adequately show the relevance of conditioning in re-initiated drug-taking, it must be demonstrated that opiate-seeking behavior will increase in *post-dependent* animals in the presence of the conditioned stimuli.

(2) Conditioned opiate effects: In the previous section we discussed the fact that stimuli paired with nalorphine in physically dependent animals can acquire the ability to elicit at least certain aspects of the opiate-withdrawal syndrome. In this section we will review the data showing that stimuli associated with opiate administration can acquire the ability to elicit some of the actions of opiates. The first report of a conditioned opiate effect was that of Collins and Tatum [7]. These investigators accidentally discovered an interesting conditioned effect in the process of studying the effects of daily injections of morphine on the dog. They found that after seven or eight daily injections, salivation and emesis, originally seen only after morphine administration, began to occur when the experimenter merely entered the room in which the dogs were housed. Subsequently, Kleitman and Crisler [26] confirmed these findings and systematically studied the conditioning and extinction of salivation with morphine as the unconditioned stimulus.

In 1964 Thompson and Schuster [46] investigated the ability of a stimulus paired with morphine reinforcement to alleviate some of the behavioral disruptions seen during withdrawal. In this experiment monkeys were conditioned on a complex multiple-reinforcement schedule to obtain food and to avoid electric shocks. In addition, the animals could self-administer intravenous morphine every 6 hours. When the opportunity to self-administer morphine was removed, the animals went into withdrawal and showed a progressive deterioration of their food- and shock-reinforced behaviors. Allowing the animals to self-administer one injection of morphine promptly returned these behaviors to baseline levels. In a replication of this study the animals were given saline (rather than morphine) accompanied by all the stimuli previously associated with morphine reinforcement. Although no morphine was administered, there was nevertheless a temporary recovery of the food-reinforced and shock-avoidance behaviors. Thus the alleviation of withdrawal by morphine became conditioned to the stimuli previously associated with morphine reinforcement. More recently Roffman, Reddy, and Lal [34] reported on the reversal or prevention of morphine-withdrawal hypothermia in rats by stimuli previously associated with morphine administration.

These experiments demonstrate that stimuli previously associated with opiates can acquire, through classical conditioning, the ability to elicit certain opiate effects. This may in fact be the mechanism underlying conditioned reinforcement. Regardless of the mechanism, however, several investigators have shown that stimuli associated with morphine reinforcement can come to act as conditioned reinforcers. Schuster and Thompson [39] reported an apparent conditioned reinforcing effect of a light which had been presented during intravenously delivered morphine reinforcement to the rhesus monkey. McGuire [29] attempted to establish a flashing light as a conditioned reinforcer by pairing it once daily with a noncontingent administration of morphine. Using the number of responses on a single extinction test as the primary measure of a conditioned reinforcing effect, McGuire failed to find a significant difference between animals experiencing pairings and controls. More recently, however, a very brief report has appeared indicating that similar procedures for establishing conditioned reinforcers have been successful [10a]. Schuster and Woods [42] investigated the conditioned reinforcing effects of a light previously paired with morphine reinforcement in the rhesus monkey. This experiment showed that the light had acquired conditioned reinforcing properties, as indicated by its ability to maintain higher response rates in extinction. Of great theoretical and practical significance was the finding that this conditioned reinforcing effect remained even after an interpolated 20-day drug abstinence. Thus the conditioned reinforcing effect was independent of the organism's state of physical dependence.

Conditioned reinforcement in rats ingesting morphine orally has also been recently reported [44]. This study showed that rats who had orally ingested "bitter" morphine solutions drank more of the bitter quinine solution than rats who had never ingested morphine. Since bitterness had been associated with morphine reinforcement, it had acquired conditioned reinforcing properties.

These findings are extremely important in understanding the apparent functional autonomy of ritualistic behavior of the experienced drug addict. The chain of behaviors involves hustling for money, purchasing the drug, preparing the drug, and finally taking (either orally or parenterally) the drug; all these, clearly, have stimulus feedback which can acquire conditioned reinforcing properties because they are associated, at least intermittently, with the primary reinforcing actions of the drug. Since such conditioned reinforcers are not dependent upon the presence of physical dependence, they may survive detoxification periods in hospitals or prisons and thus contribute to "relapse" to opiate use.

CONCLUSIONS

For several reasons the conceptualization of the problem of drug abuse in the context of behavioral analysis is more than an academic exercise. In contrast to traditional approaches to drug abuse in which the source of difficulty is placed within the individual, the behavior analyst stresses the importance of the control of an individual's behavior by environmental contingencies. This has tremendous implications for treatment programs, which, to be maximally effective, must consider all the environmental factors maintaining an individual's self-administration of drugs. Only when these are analyzed can a rational program of behavioral modification be designed and implemented. The present review has indicated at least some of the sources of control which maintain self-administration behavior and, as well, has suggested several classes of variables the manipulation of which can decrease the frequency of occurrence of this behavior.

REFERENCES

1. Azrin, N. H., & Holz, W. C. Punishment. In W. F. Honig (Ed.), *Operant behavior: Areas of research and application*. New York: Appleton-Century-Crofts, 1966.
2. Azzi, R., Fix, D. S. R., Keller, F. S., & Rocha e Silva, M. Exteroceptive control of response under delayed reinforcement. *Journal of Experimental Analysis of Behavior*, 7, 159–162, 1964.
3. Balster, R. L., Johanson, C. E., & Schuster, C. R. The evaluation of reinforcement efficacy of psychoactive drugs: II. Choice procedures. *Psychopharmacologia*, in preparation.
4. Balster, R. L., & Schuster, C. R. Fixed-interval schedule of cocaine reinforcement: Effect of dose and infusion duration. *Journal of Experimental Analysis of Behavior*, 20, 119–129, 1973.
5. Balster, R. L., Schuster, C. R., & Wilson, M. C. The substitution of opiate analgesics in monkeys maintained on cocaine self-administration. Paper presented at the 33rd annual meeting of the Committee on Problems of Drug Dependence, NAS-NRC, Toronto, February 1971.
6. Claghorn, J. F., Ordy, J. M., & Nagy, A. Spontaneous opiate addiction in rhesus monkeys. *Science*, 149, 440–441, 1965.
7. Collins, K. H., & Tatum, A. L. A conditioned reflex established by chronic morphine poisoning. *Amer. J. Physiol.*, 74, 15, 1925.
8. Collins, R. J., & Weeks, J. R. Relative potency of codeine, methadone and dihydromorphinone to morphine in self-maintained addict rats. *Naunynschmiedebergs Arch. Exp. Path. Pharmak.*, 249, 509–514, 1965.
9. Collins, R. J., & Weeks, J. R. Lack of effect of dexoxadrol in self-maintained morphine dependence in rats. *Psychopharmacologia*, 11, 289–292, 1967.
10. Davis, W. M., & Smith, S. G. Alpha-methyltyrosine to prevent self-administration of morphine and amphetamine. *Current Therapeutic Research*, 14, 814–819, 1972.
10a. Davis, W. M., Smith, S. G., & Crowder, W. F. Morphine based conditioned reinforcement. Paper presented at the Fifth International Congress on Pharmacology, San Francisco, July 1972.
11. Deneau, G., Yanagita, T., & Seevers, M. H. Self-administration of psychoactive substances in the monkey. A measure of psychological dependence. *Psychopharmacologia*, 16, 30–48, 1969.
12. Ferster, C. B., & Hammer, C. Variables determining the effects of delay in reinforcement. *J. Exp. Anal. Behav.*, 8, 243–254, 1965.
13. Ferster, C. B., & Skinner, B. F. *Schedules of reinforcement*. New York: Appleton-Century-Crofts, 1957.
14. Findley, J. P., Robinson, W. W., & Peregrino, L. Addiction to secobarbital and chlordiazepoxide in the rhesus monkey by means of a self-infusion preference procedure. *Psychopharmacologia*, 26, 93–114, 1972.
15. Fink, M. Narcotic antagonists in opiate dependence. *Science*, 169, 1005–1006, 1970.
16. Goldberg, S. R., & Schuster, C. R. Conditioned suppression by a stimulus associated with nalorphine in morphine-dependent monkeys. *J. Exp. Anal. Behav.*, 10, 235–242, 1967.
17. Goldberg, S. R., & Schuster, C. R. Conditioned nalorphine-induced abstinence changes: Persistence in post morphine-dependent monkeys. *J. Exp. Anal. Behav.*, 14, 33–46, 1970.

18. Goldberg, S. R., Woods, J. H., & Schuster, C. R. Morphine: Conditioned increases in self-administration in rhesus monkeys. *Science*, 166, 1306-1307, 1969.
19. Goldberg, S. R., Woods, J. H., & Schuster, C. R. Nalorphine-induced changes in morphine self-administration in rhesus monkeys. *Journal of Pharmacology and Experimental Therapeutics*, 176, 464-471, 1971.
20. Goldberg, S. R., Hoffmeister, F., & Schlichting, U. U. Morphine antagonists: Modification of behavioral effects by morphine dependence. In J. M. Singh, L. H. Miller, & H. Lal (Eds.), *Drug Addiction*. Vol. 1. *Experimental pharmacology*. Mt. Kisco, New York: Futura Pub. Co., 1972.
21. Hoffmeister, F., & Schlichting, U. U. Reinforcing properties of some opiates and opioids in rhesus monkeys with histories of cocaine and codeine self-administration. *Psychopharmacologia*, 13, 220-227, 1972.
22. Irwin, S., & Seevers, M. H. Comparative study of regular and N-allylnormorphine induced withdrawal in monkeys addicted to morphine, 6-methylhydromorphine, dromoran, methadone and ketobemidone. *Journal of Pharmacology and Experimental Therapeutics*, 106, 397, 1952.
23. Jaffe, J. H. Narcotic analgesics. In L. S. Goodman & A. Gilman (Eds.), *The pharmacological basis of therapeutics*. New York: MacMillan, 1970.
24. Johanson, C. Choice of cocaine by rhesus monkeys as a function of dosage. *Proceedings of the 79th Annual Convention of the American Psychological Association*, 751-752, 1971.
25. Jones, B. E., & Prada, J. A. Relapse to morphine use in dog. *Psychopharmacologia* 1973, in press.
26. Kleitman, N. & Crisler, G. A quantitative study of a salivary-conditioned reflex. *Am. J. Physiol.*, 79, 571-614, 1927.
27. Kumar, R., Steinberg, H., & Stolerman, I. P. Inducing a preference for morphine in rats without premedication. *Nature*, 218, 564-565, 1968.
28. Martin, W. R., Gorodetzky, C. W., & McClane, T. K. An experimental study in the treatment of narcotic addicts with cyclazocine. *Clinical Pharmacology and Therapeutics*, 7, 455-465, 1966.
29. McGuire, L. E. Reinforcing effects of intravenously infused morphine and 1-amphetamine. Unpublished doctoral dissertation, University of Mississippi, 1966.
30. Nichols, J. R. How opiates change behavior. *Scientific American*, 212, 80-88, 1965.
31. Nichols, J. R. Morphine as a reinforcing agent: Laboratory studies of its capacity to change behavior. In A. Wikler (Ed.), *The addictive states*. Pro. of the Assoc. for Res. in Nervous and Mental Disease. Baltimore: Williams & Wilkins, 1968.
32. Nichols, J. R., & Hsiao, S. Addictive liability of albino rats: Breeding for quantitative differences in morphine drinking. *Science*, 157, 561-563, 1967.
33. Pickens, R., & Thompson, T. Reinforcement by stimulant drugs. *Proceedings of the 76th Annual Convention of the American Psychological Association*, 1968.
34. Roffman, M., Reddy, C., & Lal, H. Alleviation of morphine-withdrawal symptoms by conditional stimuli: Possible explanation for "drug hunger" and "relapse." In J. M. Singh, L. H. Miller, & H. Lal (Eds.), *Drug Addiction*. Vol. 1. *Experimental pharmacology*. Mt. Kisco, New York: Futura Pub. Co., 1972.
35. Schlichting, U. U., Goldberg, S. R., Wuttke, W., & Hoffmeister, F. D-amphetamine self-administration by rhesus monkeys with different self-administration histories. *Proceedings of the European Society for the Study of Drug Toxicity, 1970*. Excerpta Medica International Congress Series, 220, 62-69, 1971.
36. Schuster, C. R. Psychological approaches to opiate dependence and self-administration by laboratory animals. *Federation Proceedings*, 29, 2-5, 1970.
37. Schuster, C. R., & Johanson, C. E. The use of animal models for the study of drug abuse. In *Research advances in alcohol and drug problems*. New York: Wiley, 1973, in press.

38. Schuster, C. R., Smith, B. B., & Jaffe, J. H. Drug abuse in heroin users: An experimental study of self-administration of methadone, codeine, pentazocine. *Arch. Gen. Psychiatry*, **24**, 359-362, 1971.

39. Schuster, C. R., & Thompson, T. A technique for studying self-administration of opiates in rhesus monkeys. Presented at the 25th annual meeting of the Committee on the Problems of Drug Dependence, NRC–NAS, 1963.

40. Schuster, C. R., & Thompson, T. Self-administration of and behavioral dependence on drugs. *Annual Review of Pharmacology*, **9**, 483-502, 1969.

41. Schuster, C. R., & Villareal, J. E. The experimental analysis of opioid dependence. In D. H. Efron (Ed.), *Psychopharmacology: A review of progress, 1957-1967*. Washington, D.C.: U.S. Government Printing Office, 1968.

42. Schuster, C. R., & Woods, J. H. The conditioned reinforcing effects of stimuli associated with morphine reinforcement. *International Journal of the Addictions*, **3**, 223-230, 1968.

43. Skinner, B. F. *The behavior of organisms*. New York: Appleton-Century-Crofts, 1938.

44. Stolerman, I. P., & Kumar, R. Secondary reinforcement in opioid dependence. In J. M. Singh, L. H. Miller, & H. Lal (Eds.), *Drug addiction*. Vol. 1. *Experimental pharmacology*. Mt. Kisco, New York: Futura Pub. Co., 1972.

45. Thompson, T. Drugs as reinforcers: Experimental addiction. *Int. J. Addictions*, **3**, 199-206, 1968.

45a. Thompson. T., & Pickens, R. Behavioral variables influencing drug self-administration. In R. T. Harris, W. M. McIsaac, and C. R. Schuster (Eds.), *Drug Dependence*. Houston, Texas: Univ. of Texas Press, 1970.

46. Thompson, T., & Schuster, C. R. Morphine self-administration, food-reinforced and avoidance behaviors in rhesus monkeys. *Psychopharmacologia*, **5**, 87-94, 1964.

47. Thompson, T., & Schuster, C. R. *Behavioral pharmacology*. New Jersey: Prentice-Hall, 1968.

48. Weeks, J. R. Experimental morphine addiction: Method for autonomic intravenous injections in unrestrained rats. *Science*, **138**, 143-144, 1962.

49. Weeks, J. R., & Collins, R. J. Factors affecting voluntary morphine intake in self-maintained addicted rats. *Psychopharmacologia*, **6**, 267-279, 1964.

50. Woods, J. H., & Schuster, C. R. Reinforcement properties of morphine, cocaine, and SPA as a function of unit dose. *International Journal of the Addictions*, **3**, 231-237, 1968.

51. Woods, J. H., & Schuster, C. R. Opiates as reinforcing stimuli. In T. Thompson & R. Pickens (Eds.), *Stimulus properties of drugs*. New York: Appleton-Century-Crofts, 1971.

SOCIAL AND POLITICAL INFLUENCES ON ADDICTION RESEARCH

David F. Musto
Yale University

Narcotics use and control in the United States have a lengthy and complex history. Although this history cannot be directly applied to the present, some connections between social and political attitudes and addiction research are more clearly seen in retrospect. These examples may have relevance to our present debate on narcotic research. In the past, at least, the intense political significance accorded narcotic use impelled research into certain directions, gave unusual interpretations to research findings, and denied the existence of evidence which conflicted with partisan viewpoints. When narcotics are a subject of current controversy, it is difficult to disentangle the many motives and events which encompass it, but by looking at the past we can isolate some of the nonscientific forces which have appropriated or affected research. Naturally, in this brief paper detailed descriptions will have to be sacrificed so that broad patterns can be sketched [9].

In reviewing past research there are two aspects to consider. The first is the existence of a generally accepted social or scientific background against which research may be conducted. The second is the transition or crisis between periods of general agreement. In at least one such crisis, which occurred about 1920, research became sharply divided with respect to social control of drug abuse, especially opiate addiction [7]. When immersed in a general cultural tradition, almost all research of a given era continues under assumptions which to a later generation may appear arbitrary, while in times of partisan debate research reports can become the object of such fierce passions that a national program of drug control can depend on a narrow scientific issue. In the history of American narcotic control, widely assumed beliefs about the goals and objects of research and the use of research in partisan debate have deeply influenced the course of narcotics investigations and the official sanction of research activity.

Understandably, an era's social attitudes are very powerful determinants of what drugs are considered dangerous and in what way, regardless of more objective criteria. These attitudes also define which goals of research are politically significant—whether the purpose should be to control violence, combat moral degeneration, redress loss of productivity or damage to the environment. Thus one of the most frequently used arguments for liquor prohibition was based on elaborate scientific studies which estimated to what degree alcohol use decreased personal and national productivity. And control of barbiturates was until recently neglected, while smoking opium, linked earlier in the century to feared, alien Chinese, aroused furious opposition and denunciation.

The assumption of a close association between cocaine and Southern blacks is another example of how dominant social attitudes can create a stereotyped drug menace. At the turn of this century sexual assaults and other kinds of anti-white hostility were attributed to the use of cocaine by blacks, until the connection between the drug and this minority group became an accepted cliché [12]. It is significant that this association came at the peak of black disenfranchisement and lynchings. Of course, the drug's reputed link with racially motivated unrest made any form of availability intolerable except for limited medical usage. Probably the association with a feared minority assisted the almost total prohibition of cocaine at the same time that fewer and looser restrictions were being placed on morphine.

Marijuana is a more recent example of drugs so closely connected with violence that no form of licensed regulation could be permitted. During the 1930s marijuana was almost universally thought to release inhibitions to violence and was often said to incite the most vicious crimes [8]. Its wide acceptance as a destroyer of inhibitions contrasts with present descriptions of its behavioral effects. Among various possible explanations for this change in clinical experience, one probable factor would be the cultural expectation of violence from marijuana use—an expectation which affected both the investigator and the user. In recent years marijuana's reputation as the weed of evil has often been ascribed to a clever plot of the Federal Bureau of Narcotics and occasionally to some other conspiracy. Yet at the time of the Marijuana Tax Act (1937) the most widely held medical opinion was that the drug released inhibitions and thereby led to violence. Harshly regulative control of smoking opium, cocaine, and marijuana, then, are examples of how the social milieu shaped public response and determined the relevance of research.

Generally accepted forms of scientific explanation can similarly reflect assumptions which in later years seem overapplied. For example, in the course of extensive research on addiction before 1920, the most common assumption, and one which underlay several "cures," was that morphine or any other opiate stimulated antibody or antitoxin production in the user's body [7]. Repeatedly, antitoxins or antibodies were claimed to be demonstrated in animals made opiate-dependent; it was also reported that these substances could be transferred to normal animals with appropriate effect. This popular explanation was not seriously questioned until it became a key issue in a bitter and politically colored battle in the United States about the time of World War I.

Before discussing the collision between immunochemical hypotheses and later dominant views on the control of social deviance in the United States, I would like to give one more example of a broad and, at the time, widely accepted assumption on which much of addiction research operated for a decade or so after 1920. This is the belief that the fundamental flaw in the addict is psychological and not biochemical. This view is represented best in the papers written in the 1920s by a leading American expert on addiction, Dr. Lawrence Kolb, Sr. In these early papers Dr. Kolb was quite explicit in arguing that only the psychopath could become addicted. Although he later modified these beliefs, he also thought that the sensual pleasure of opiates could not be experienced except by a psychopath; a normal person would experience only relief from pain [5]. In 1920 an AMA committee on addiction advocated the "newer psychology" for the ultimate cure of the addict through sublimation of his lower instincts [1]. Thus the advent of dynamic psychology, which located deviance within the personality of the individual and his early character formation, arrived at a most convenient time in the crisis over the immunological explanation of addiction. The dispute turned on the wisdom of permitting addiction maintenance. Those favoring the immunochemical explanation of "addiction-disease" based their argument for addiction maintenance on the presence of antibodies or antitoxins. They argued that providing an opiate would counteract the immune substance and restore the addict to a normal state [2]. On the other hand, the progressive leadership of the AMA and a majority of the Supreme Court, to name two substantial opponents, believed maintenance of addiction to be extremely poor public policy and, in fact, disastrous for the social harmony of the nation. In this way a scientific question, the presence of antibodies, became a matter of the greatest import in a public debate over the best way to control what was thought by many institutions to be a grave threat to national security.

Now let us turn to the transition—from that period of confidence in the biochemical explanation of addiction to one of emphasis on dynamic psychology. This shift in respectable opinion occurred within a relatively brief time, about 3 or 4 years, and the final battle, during which the adherents of maintenance were scattered, took perhaps a year. This brief interspace suggests how uncomfortable it is for both scientists and bureaucrats to tolerate indecision and frustrations over a major social question. The outcome of this medico-political crisis was in effect the outlawing of what had been a respectable approach to addiction and the harassment and jailing of those who persisted in practicing maintenance either as a measure to employ until a cure could be found, or on grounds that the disease was incurable and treatable only in this way. The policy implication of certain research claims, that antibodies to morphine existed in the addict, was accepted by both camps as implying that maintenance was justified. Some respected clinicians were led into intellectual contortions as they attempted to blunt the impact of such research. Finally, the personal motivations of those who professed belief in immunological claims were questioned, and many were considered avaricious, evil, or simply troublemakers.

Therefore, the crisis in 1919, the crucial year for this change in scientific outlook, was over the implications drawn from research for the social control of deviance. Psychological explanations, particularly those which ascribed to environment the formation of character, were favored—seeming to imply that addiction was a habit that could be corrected through psychological treatment. The anti-maintainers did not believe that antibodies or antitoxins to opiates existed, and they conducted some apparently accurate research to prove this contention [11]. Another favored claim of pro-maintainers, that abrupt opiate withdrawal would lead to many deaths among addicts, was also strongly denied. This fight became so intense that by 1921 the Surgeon General of the Public Health Service considered the phrase "physiological balance" to be so "controversial" that he advised, confidentially, that it be omitted from a discussion of narcotic treatment [3].

Why this debate over a question to be settled in the laboratory? The controversy can be largely ascribed to a general fear around 1919 in the United States that the nation was in mortal danger from politically deviant domestic minorities. National and local responses to threats from the IWW, Bolsheviks and socialists are known well enough to be noted here merely by reference [6]. Addicts were lumped into this collection of domestic threats and were confronted by various social institutions as vigorously as was the IWW. Any proposal to maintain addicts in their drug supply was taken to mean the preservation of a group which was held responsible for much of the crime in New York City and for a wave of violent crimes said to be sweeping the nation; a group, in the opinion of Mayor John Hylan of New York City, linked with anarchists and bombers.

The battle, then, was over opposing implications of scientific research for social policy. One set of findings was soon considered almost "un-American" and further research in the 1920s was devoted to disproving any existence of immunological entities in the blood as a result of opiate ingestion [4]. Another favorite target of research was disproving the specific cures which were based on the immunological hypothesis [10]. The conflict at its origin lined up the AMA leadership and federal antinarcotic agencies on the same side; it was not, at the time, a dispute neatly dividing doctors from policemen.

In looking back on that bitter dispute of 50 years ago, the problem becomes apparent for preserving open research in addiction: namely, that political closure can be imposed on a subject when major questions are yet to be answered. Research in addiction has paid a price for its close involvement with questions of deviance control.

In the 1920s and for decades thereafter a view of addiction representing one aspect of the question was enshrined in law. Yet, in stating this, I am not arguing that the viewpoint which became law was wrong; rather, I would argue that political pressure led to a situation in which dissident research became less likely. If the state of knowledge about addiction had been like that about smallpox, where compulsory vaccination can be supported with considerable confidence, the institutionalization of one point of view would have been more acceptable. But since this is not the case with addiction, political considerations which restrict possible research are undesirable.

A similar crisis and result occurred in the 1930s in the case of marijuana, when a consensus of its link with violence became part of the law and subsequent conflicting research was felt as an embarrassment or even evilly motivated. The FBN, for example, felt deep disappointment with some medical studies that questioned the Bureau's strong anti-marijuana stand, almost as if the investigator's had betrayed the Bureau's provision of drugs and other assistance. Research involving drugs which have or are alleged to have effect on behavior has profound political implications which threaten to interfere with responsible scientific investigation. As our examination of the crisis in 1919 suggests, research options in addiction can become restricted in as short a period as one year. An additional problem of politically significant research is that the genuine beliefs of most scientists at one time may, with all good intentions, become encased in law and enforced by legal institutions for a very long time.

Although the political power of scientific investigators is small when compared to the larger social and political forces which shape national response to deviance, perhaps recalling the vicissitudes of the past may help keep open avenues of research which may not fit in with contemporary political judgments.

REFERENCES

1. American Medical Association. Report of the committee on the narcotic drug situation in the United States. *JAMA, 74,* 1324–1328, 1920.
2. Bishop, E. S. *The narcotic drug problem.* New York: Macmillan, 1920.
3. Cumming, H. S. (Surgeon General of the U.S. Public Health Service) Letter dated February 12, 1921, to Oscar Dowling, President of the Louisiana State Board of Health. Records of the Public Health Service, File No. 2123, National Archives, Washington, D.C.
4. Karr, W. G., Light, A. B., & Torrance, E. G. Opium addiction. IV. Blood of human addict during administration of morphine. *Arch. Int. Med., 43,* 684–690, 1929.
5. Kolb, L. Pleasure and deterioration from narcotic addiction. *Mental Hygiene, 9,* 699–724, 1925.
6. Murray, R. K. *Red scare: A study of national hysteria, 1919-1920.* Minneapolis: University of Minnesota Press, 1955.
7. Musto, D. F., The American antinarcotic movement: clinical research and public policy. *Clinical Research, 19,* 601–605, 1971.
8. Musto, D. F. The marihuana tax act of 1937. *Arch. of Gen. Psychiat., 26,* 101–108, 1972.

9. Musto, D. F. *The American disease: Origins of narcotic control.* New Haven: Yale University Press, 1973.
10. New York City Mayor's Committee on Drug Addiction: Report. *American Journal of Psychiatry,* 10, 433-538, 1930.
11. Pellini, E. J., & Greenfield, A. D. Narcotic drug addiction: I. The formation of protective substances against morphin. *Arch. Int. Med.,* 26, 279-292, 1920.
12. Williams, E. H. Negro cocaine 'fiends' are a new Southern menace. *New York Times,* February 8, 1914, Section V, p. 12.

SOME BIOCHEMICAL ASPECTS OF MORPHINE TOLERANCE AND PHYSICAL DEPENDENCE[1]

E. Leong Way
University of California School of Medicine

Pharmacologists readily recognize that drug dependence is principally a psychiatric and social problem, and that the core is the person rather than the drug. Nonetheless, pharmacologic considerations strongly dictate whether or not a substance will become abused. In addition to the immediate psychotropic effects of a particular drug on mood and perception, its potential for abuse may be greatly enhanced by the development of tolerance and physical dependence. This is especially true for heroin and other morphine surrogates. The development of tolerance and physical dependence following their repeated administration is a strong reinforcing factor which leads to compulsive use. It is not surprising, then, that pharmacologists have been engrossed by the ability of morphine to effect tolerance and physical dependence and have sought to explain these two properties.

Dr. Cochin, in his chapter, discusses in some detail the general theories on tolerance and physical dependence. He has also made my task much easier by citing the various experimental approaches used by other investigators. Since we have had occasion to review this field as well, and since these writings have been published or are in press [55, 56, 59], my discussion here will be limited primarily to the work being carried out in our laboratory.

[1] The studies cited from our laboratories were largely supported by research grants from the U.S. Department of Health, Education, and Welfare, National Institute of Mental Health (MH-17017) and the National Institutes of Health (RG-01839). The work was mostly carried out by my colleagues and collaborators Drs. H. H. Loh, I. K. Ho, H. N. Bhargava, E. T. Iwamoto, E. Wei, and R. J. Hitzemann, and I am grateful to them for their comments and suggestions.

In brief, our studies indicate that it is possible to dissociate selectively with pharmacologic tools the processes involved in the immediate pharmacologic effects of morphine from those which might be connected with the development of tolerance and dependence. We have obtained evidence that the acute pharmacologic responses to morphine can be modified greatly without significantly altering tolerance and physical dependence development. On the other hand, we have also found that the development of tolerance and dependence can be blocked without modifying the acute pharmacologic action of morphine. Evidence has been obtained, moreover, suggesting that the development of the tolerant-dependent state can be accelerated. We conclude from our results that the synthesis of some macromolecule, distinct from the receptor protein at the morphine effector site, is being increasingly modified as tolerance and physical dependence develop. I shall describe some of the work carried out in our laboratory by excerpting from some of our original publications and reviews.

ASSESSMENT OF TOLERANCE AND PHYSICAL DEPENDENCE

In our laboratory we use the mouse and rat as a model; the classic effects of morphine such as analgesia, tolerance, and physical dependence can easily be demonstrated in both species. By modifying the subcutaneous morphine pellet implantation procedure originally reported by Huidobro and Maggiolo [30], we have been able to produce rapidly a high degree of tolerance and physical dependence, and maximal effects are observable within 3 days [58, 60].

Tolerance to morphine is measured by noting the increase in the amount of the drug (morphine AD50) to produce analgesia as measured by the classic tail-flick antinociceptive procedure. Physical dependence on morphine can be assessed after abrupt withdrawal by removing the pellet or by precipitating withdrawal with the narcotic antagonist, naloxone. The withdrawal signs after abrupt precipitated withdrawal are much slower in onset, are less intense, and persist longer. In the mouse, the most characteristic sign of precipitated withdrawal is stereotyped jumping. The degree of dependence on morphine can be quantified by estimating the amount of naloxone (ED50) to precipitate the response. An inverse relationship exists between the two parameters; the higher the degree of dependence, the lower the naloxone ED50 [27, 58, 60]. Degree of dependence can also be assessed after abrupt withdrawal by following body weight after pellet removal; dependent animals lose considerable body weight during abstinence [27, 28, 49].

BLOCKADE OF TOLERANCE AND PHYSICAL DEPENDENCE DEVELOPMENT BY INHIBITORS OF PROTEIN SYNTHESIS

The possibility that either morphine tolerance or physical dependence, or both, may result from modification of a macromolecule in the brain has been considered by several laboratories. In the studies described by Dr. Cochin (this volume), inhibitors of protein synthesis were noted to block the development of tolerance to morphine. In our laboratory, we have found that the development of physical dependence on and tolerance to morphine can be inhibited in the mouse by the concomitant administration of cycloheximide [37].

We have also noted that the inhibiting effect by cycloheximide on tolerance development was attained without an alteration in the analgetic response to morphine. As Figure 1 shows, the repeated injection of morphine resulted in considerable tolerance development; the dose of morphine required to produce analgesia in this group increased several fold. On the other hand, the concurrent

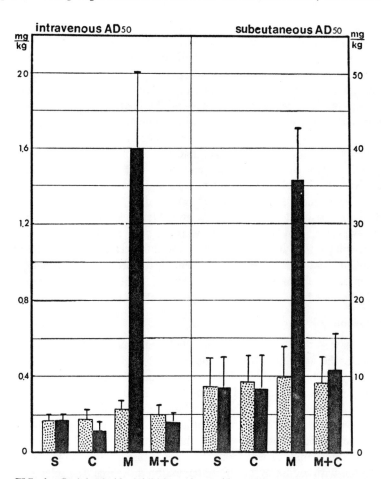

FIG. 1. Cycloheximide inhibition of morphine tolerance development as measured by the analgetic response to morphine before (stippled bars) and after (black bars) repeated daily treatment for 21 days with: saline (S); cycloheximide (C); morphine (M); and morphine and cycloheximide (M + C). The brackets denote the S. E. (*From Loh, Shen, and Way*, [37] *with permission.*)

administration of cycloheximide with morphine did not result in an elevation of the morphine AD50. The analgetic response of the latter group was not significantly different from that of the group injected repeatedly with either saline or cycloheximide alone. Moreover, the treatments with cycloheximide prevented the development of physical dependence, as evidenced by an inhibition of the naloxone-precipitated withdrawal jumping response. It was suggested as a consequence that the protein (or macromolecule) involved in tolerance and/or physical dependence could not be the receptor protein involved in mediating the acute effect of morphine, but was rather some other macromolecule with a more rapid turnover rate [37].

POSSIBLE ROLE OF NEUROTRANSMITTERS

Inasmuch as the inhibitors of protein synthesis have widespread effects, the task of identifying the macromolecule possibly involved with the development of morphine tolerance and dependence is rather formidable. To understand the processes involved, we attempted to assess the contributory role of the putative neurotransmitters in these conditions by manipulating their functional state in the CNS. Various pharmacologic tools have been utilized to affect as selectively as possible the synthesis, storage, release, or degradation of acetylcholine, dopamine, norepinephrine, and serotonin, and the consequence of such maneuvers on the tolerant-dependent state and on the development of tolerance to and dependence on morphine were evaluated.

On the basis of the data now available, it appears that acetylcholine, norepinephrine, and dopamine may participate in the mediation of acute pharmacologic responses to morphine as well as certain withdrawal signs of the dependent state; however, they seem less directly concerned with the development of tolerance to and physical dependence on morphine. Our conclusions are based on the following observations for each substance.

Acetylcholine

We have confirmed the early literature that cholinesterase inhibition augments the analgetic effect of morphine, but we have also found that this process is still functional to the same relative degree in animals rendered tolerant to morphine. In mice rendered tolerant by pellet implantation, as evidenced by a several-fold elevation of the morphine AD50, administration of either physostigmine or DFP to the tolerant animals also resulted in a lowering of the morphine AD50. However, since the relative change effected by either cholinesterase inhibitor was about the same as that observed in nontolerant mice implanted with a dummy pellet containing no morphine, the tolerant state was not modified by this treatment. Moreover, development of tolerance was also not affected. The administration of DFP prior to morphine pellet implantation resulted in a lowering of the morphine AD50 comparable to that obtained in mice that had been previously rendered maximally tolerant by implantation. The ratio of the morphine AD50 of tolerant over nontolerant animals receiving DFP was nearly identical with the ratio in tolerant and nontolerant animals without DFP treatment. We interpreted this to mean that cholinesterase inhibition does not affect materially the development of tolerance to morphine [5].

Our studies indicate that cholinesterase inhibition may modify the morphine-dependent state but not the development of dependence. In mice rendered dependent by pellet implantation, pronounced inhibition of naloxone-precipitated withdrawal jumping was evidenced by an over-20-fold elevation of the naloxone ED50 immediately after physostigmine or DFP treatment. However, despite the striking response elicited, the treatment did not have a significant effect on physical dependence development. When physostigmine was injected repeatedly before and during the period of morphine pellet implantation, 24 hours after the last administration, its effects on naloxone-precipitated withdrawal jumping as measured by the naloxone ED50 were negative. Secondly, DFP failed to inhibit body weight loss after abrupt withdrawal was initiated by removal of the morphine pellet. Had DFP produced a general inhibitory effect on morphine dependence development, it should have prevented the loss in weight which occurred upon pellet removal [5].

Catecholamines

Our results also suggest that the catecholamines participate in some of the acute pharmacologic responses of morphine and in the end response of some withdrawal signs of the dependent state, but do not appear to be primarily involved with either tolerance or physical dependence development. This conclusion rests primarily on the results of our studies with 6-hydroxydopamine (6-OHDA). The compound, 6-OHDA, was found to effect reduction of the catecholamines in the peripheral nervous system [44] by causing acute degeneration of adrenergic nerve endings [52]. More recently, it has been reported to effect a prolonged reduction in the brain concentrations of norepinephrine and dopamine but not serotonin after intraventricular injection, and it was suggested that 6-OHDA also effected selective destruction of the catecholamine neurons in the Central Nervous System [6, 54].

Our studies with 6-OHDA suggest that norepinephrine may be concerned in morphine antinociception, but the experiments in mice rendered tolerant by morphine pellet implantation indicate that 6-OHDA does not affect tolerance development. The lowering of brain norepinephrine and dopamine effected by 6-OHDA pretreatment was accompanied by a decrease in analgetic response to morphine not only in the nontolerant mouse but in the tolerant one as well. As shown in Figure 2, the morphine AD50 was increased by 6-OHDA pretreatment in both tolerant and nontolerant animals, and the relative increase for each group was approximately the same. We interpret this to mean that 6-OHDA affects the acute response to morphine but not the process that is primarily involved in initiating the development of tolerance to morphine [16].

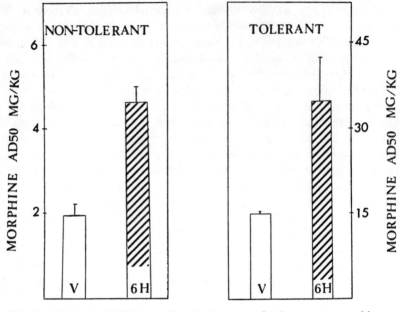

FIG. 2. Effect of 6-OHDA on the development of tolerance to morphine as measured by the analgetic response to morphine. The morphine AD50 was determined before and after the animals were rendered tolerant by morphine pellet implantation. 6-OHDA (6H) or vehicle (V) was injected intracerebrally 2 days before pellet implantation. (*From Table 1, Friedler et al.*[16], *with permission.*)

Apart from the apparent negative effects of the catecholamines on morphine tolerance and dependence development, there are some interesting acute effects morphine elicits on bioamine metabolism that can be correlated with pharmacologic events.

In an attempt to elucidate the possible mechanism by which morphine may interact with norepinephrine, we initiated a study on the effect of morphine on brain catecholamine dynamics [35]. Previous studies with ^{14}C-tyrosine showed that morphine increased the incorporation of the labeled precursor into brain catecholamines [12, 50]. Using ^{14}C-tyrosine, we confirmed that there was, indeed, increased catecholamine synthesis after an analgetic dose of morphine; in addition, we found evidence that this was due mainly to increased ^{14}C-tyrosine brain uptake. The increased catecholamine synthesis was accompanied by a preferential release of norepinephrine and, as a consequence, we suggested that the release of newly synthesized norepinephrine may be coupled to the neurochemical events associated with morphine antinociception [35].

In additional studies, we found evidence that the stereotyped jumping which occurs in morphine-dependent mice or rats after abrupt or naloxone-precipitated withdrawal may depend upon a sudden elevation of brain dopamine levels. When naloxone was given to mice and rats rendered dependent on morphine by pellet implantation, brain levels of dopamine, but not those of norepinephrine and 5-HT, suddenly increased to 20 to 40% above control levels within 5 minutes coincidentally with the peak in precipitated stereotyped jumping. The increase in dopamine preceded the jumping response since it occurred also in dependent mice which were prevented from jumping by curarization. Reduction of brain catecholamines by inhibition of its synthesis with alpha-methyl-p-tyrosine partially blocked the increase in dopamine after naloxone and increased the amount of naloxone required to induce jumping. Elevation of acetylcholine by cholinesterase inhibition with physostigmine blocked the sudden rise of dopamine levels as well as the jumping response. Hence, the jumping response appears to be modulated via cholinergic-dopaminergic pathways [31] and related to, if not dependent on, a sudden elevation of brain dopamine.

Serotonin

It appeared worth while to examine the role of serotonin in the genesis of morphine tolerance and dependence for several reasons. Molecular models of morphine and 5-HT exhibit some degree of complementariness. The recent attempts to implicate serotonin in the sleep mechanisms, temperature regulation, social and sexual behavior, and pain mechanisms have made it increasingly attractive to study interactions between serotonin and morphine, since the latter compound can affect all the above functions. It has been reported also by Huidobro and his associates [29] that the administration of serotonin or its metabolic precursors attenuated the abstinence syndrome. Collier [13] proposed that an adaptive increase in the supply of receptors for a particular neurohormone may occur if morphine acts either by reducing levels of an excitatory transmitter or by occupying the receptor sites. Among the several neurohormones he considered that might oppose morphine, Collier mentioned serotonin; he also pointed out that the central effects of the serotonin precursor, 5-HTP, are similar in certain respects to the abstinence syndrome. Since the focus of research in the brain amines has shifted largely to dynamic factors that might influence the steady state, we decided to study the rate of serotonin synthesis in morphine tolerant-dependent animals.

A comparison of the turnover of brain serotonin in tolerant and nontolerant mice revealed a mean increase in tolerant animals more than double that in nontolerants [27, 48, 57]. To obtain our data, we used the pargyline method of Tozer, Neff, and Brodie [53] which involves blocking the conversion of 5-HT to 5-HIAA with the MAO-inhibitor pargyline. On the assumption that brain 5-HT is converted solely to 5-HIAA, the rate of 5-HT synthesis may be calculated from the rate of accumulation of 5-HT. We also used the probenecid procedure of Neff, Tozer, and Brodie [43] in a limited number of studies to measure the rise in 5-HIAA when the transport of 5-HIAA from the cerebral spinal fluid to blood is blocked.

Our findings with respect to morphine enhancement of brain 5-HT turnover in the tolerant-dependent state have been challenged by several laboratories using different procedures to measure 5-HT turnover [1, 10, 39], but also by one laboratory using the pargyline procedure [46]. However, our observations in the morphine tolerant-dependent mouse that increased brain serotonin turnover occurs have been amply confirmed on three strains of mice in Takemori's laboratory [40]. Moreover, Haubrich and Blake [19], using the probenecid procedure to measure brain 5-HT turnover in the rat, noted that the rate of accumulation of 5-HIAA in animals rendered tolerant to morphine by pellet implantation was considerably greater than that in nontolerant controls. Methadone also appears to increase brain 5-HT turnover [7].

The basis for the different findings has been debated [9, 20, 27]. Possibly the procedures for calculating 5-HT turnover in the normal state may not have the same validity when the animal is under the influence of a drug. Nonetheless, although the absolute values may be open to question, we consistently find evidence of an increased turnover of 5-HT after repeated injections of morphine. A recent study of the 5-HT turnover in four brain regions by the pargyline method revealed that the most pronounced change occurred in the hypothalamus and brain stem, and lesser effects were noted in the cortex and cerebellum [27]. More recently, we have compared the brain 5-HT turnover of morphine tolerant-dependent mice and nontolerant ones by the ^{3}H-tryptophan procedure [34], and we have noted a higher rate of conversion of tryptophan into 5-HT in the tolerant-dependent state. A study of the uptake of labeled tryptophan in brain showed higher specific activities for tryptophan and 5-HT in morphine tolerant-dependent mice (see Figure 3).

In findings consistent with ours, two laboratories reported independently that the rate limiting enzyme involved in serotonin synthesis is increased in the morphine-dependent rat. Azmitia et al. [2] noted an increase in tryptophan hydroxylase activity in the midbrain areas of rats given repeated injections of morphine, and a pronounced elevation was noted in the synaptosomes of the septal areas by Mandell et al. [38]. These findings are of considerable import since Schecter, Lovenberg, and Sjoerdsma [46], using a $DMPH_4$-dependent fraction prepared from whole mouse brain, were unable to find any difference in total brain tryptophan hydroxylase activity between tolerant and nontolerant mice. According to Knapp and Mandell [32], a possible explanation for the negative data is that there are two forms of tryptophan hydroxylase, a soluble and a particulate form, and only the soluble enzyme could be dependent on exogenous $DMPH_4$ since nerve endings do not take up this cofactor. Morphine does not affect the soluble form of tryptophan hydroxylase, but only the particulate form.

It is not certain whether the increased tryptophan hydroxylase activity occurring in the morphine tolerant-dependent state bears any important relationship to tolerance and physical dependence development. On the other hand, there are sufficient experimental data to suggest that serotonin may be meaningfully associated with these conditions. I will describe our results with three agents that affect the metabolic state of serotonin in CNS.

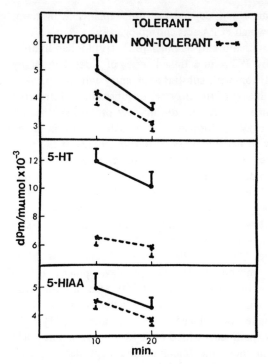

FIG. 3. Conversion of a pulse dose of ^{3}H-tryptophan into radiolabeled 5-HT and 5-HIAA in morphine tolerant and non-tolerant mice. Mice were rendered tolerant by morphine pellet implantation for 72 hours. (*From Loh, Cho, Ho, and Way* [34], *unpublished.*)

p-Chlorophenylalanine (PCPA)

PCPA has been reported to be a relatively specific and long-lasting inhibitor of 5-HT synthesis [33]. An assessment of the analgetic response to morphine in mice implanted with morphine after pretreatment with PCPA indicated that this compound reduced tolerance development to morphine. The increase in morphine AD50 resulting from morphine pellet implantation was reduced approximately one-half by PCPA. Moreover, with more prolonged administration of morphine and PCPA, evidence was obtained that development of dependence was also reduced. The naloxone ED50 for precipitated withdrawal jumping in dependent animals after PCPA was roughly doubled [27, 48, 57].

Several laboratories reported that they were unable to confirm certain aspects of our work. These differences have been discussed in a more recent publication [27]. The chief difference in experimental conditions was that we evaluated the effects of PCPA in animals which had more protracted morphine dependence. It is likely that some of the reported discrepancies concerning PCPA effects on morphine tolerance and dependence are explainable in terms of the varying mechanisms by which PCPA acts chronologically.

According to Knapp and Mandell [32], tryptophan hydroxylase appears to be influenced by PCPA in a linked series of three temporally related events, namely, competition with substrate for entry into the nerve ending, reversible competitive inhibition of the enzyme for substrate, and irreversible inhibition by incorporation into the enzyme during new protein synthesis in the cell body. The defective enzyme formed in the latter event is then transported by axoplasmic flow to nerve endings of the septal area at the rate of about 1 to 2 mm/day. Hence, in utilizing PCPA to elucidate biochemical mechanisms underlying behavioral and pharmacologic phenomena, the temporal sequence of all three mechanisms for decreasing brain 5-HT should be considered.

We have since confirmed our previous findings in the mouse and have obtained supporting evidence in the rat as well. As Figure 4 shows, in morphine pellet animals, pre- and concurrent treatment with PCPA results in a reduction of the morphine AD50 and elevation of the naloxone ED50. Furthermore, attenuation of morphine dependence development by PCPA was also demonstrated by its effect on weight loss after abrupt withdrawal. In mice rendered dependent by pellet implantation, the weight loss occurring after removal of the pellet was reduced by PCPA treatment [27].

More recent experiments with 5,6-dihydroxytryptamine (DHT) also support a role for 5-HT in morphine tolerance and dependence [38]. DHT has been reported by Baumgarten et al. [3] to destroy selectively serotonergic nerve endings. As illustrated in Figure 5, pretreatment of mice intracerebrally with a dose that effected a lowering of 5-HT by about 50% resulted in a reduction in both tolerance and dependence development, as evidenced by a decrease in the morphine AD50 and an increase in the naloxone ED50 [25].

Our experiments with tryptophan further support an associated role for 5-HT in morphine tolerance and dependence. Recent evidence by Fernstrom and Wurtman [14] suggests that the regulation of brain 5-HT synthesis may depend upon the availability of its amino acid precursor. Tryptophan was found to accelerate the development of tolerance. In experiments on mice implanted with a morphine pellet for 3 days, the relative increase in the morphine AD50 of tryptophan-treated animals was nearly 5 times that of the vehicle-treated group. No significant change in the morphine AD50 was noted between vehicle- and tryptophan-injected mice receiving a placebo implant. Similar experiments in the rat also indicated that tryptophan enhanced tolerance development to morphine [22].

In addition to accelerating morphine tolerance development, tryptophan enhanced the development of physical dependence. In mice treated with tryptophan before and daily during morphine pellet implantation, the naloxone ED50 for precipitating withdrawal jumping was approximately one-fourth that of the control group receiving saline instead of tryptophan. In the rat, similar experiments with tryptophan also resulted in a more dependent state, as

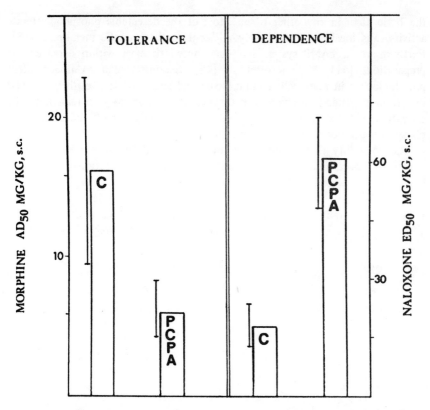

FIG. 4. PCPA inhibition of morphine tolerance and physical dependence development in the rat. The animals were rendered tolerant and dependent by morphine pellet implantation. The left panel indicates the s.c. morphine AD50 and 95% confidence limits for animals treated with either PCPA or its vehicle (C). The right panel indicates the s.c. naloxone ED50 for precipitating withdrawal jumping with and without PCPA treatment. (*From Ho, Lu, Stolman, Loh, and Way* [27], *with permission.*)

evidenced by a fourfold reduction in the naloxone ED50. Furthermore, as Figure 6 shows, the tryptophan-treated animals lost most weight when abrupt withdrawal was initiated by pellet removal. The increased weight loss effected by tryptophan was largely antagonized by PCPA. Thus, PCPA not only reduces the development of physical dependence on morphine but also blocks the accelerating effects of tryptophan on the process [22].

Adenosine 3′, 5′-Cyclic Monophosphate (cAMP)

There has been increasing evidence that cAMP may be involved in the regulation of metabolism and function in nervous tissue [18]. Its functional role in brain is still obscure, but its probable importance in synaptic transmission is suggested by the fact that the levels of adenyl cyclase, the enzyme which forms cAMP, and phosphodiesterase, which breaks it down, are 10–20 times higher in the brain than in any other tissue. Most of the detectable phosphodiesterase activity was localized immediately adjacent to the synaptic membrane [15]. Furthermore, a cAMP system has been noted to exist within nerve ending preparations [41]. Miyamoto et al. [42] demonstrated a cAMP-dependent protein kinase in mammalian brain tissue and suggested that both short- and long-term physiological changes in the nervous system may be related to the activation of cyclic nucleotide-dependent protein kinase with the consequent phosphorylation of macromolecules or histone.

The possibility that cAMP might interact with morphine was suggested by numerous reports indicating that morphine can alter the functional state of the biogenic amines, and that the latter substances can modify morphine actions. Recently, morphine was found to activate cerebral adenyl cyclase by Chou et al. [11], and centrally applied cAMP was reported to induce striking behavior alterations [17]. The mounting evidence that cyclic AMP might have a role in

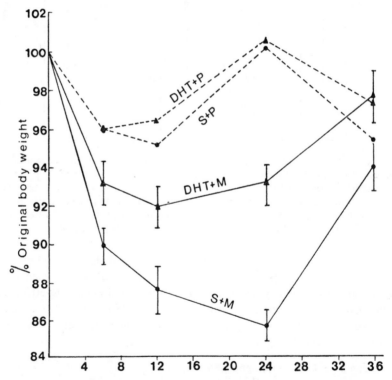

FIG. 5. DHT inhibition of physical dependence development on morphine in the mouse as indicated by mean ± S. E. body weight loss after abrupt withdrawal. Mice were rendered dependent by morphine pellet implantation for 3 days and abstinence was induced by removal of the pellet. The animals were treated with M, morphine pellet; P, placebo pellet; DHT, 5,6-dihydroxytryptamine; S, saline. *(From Ho, Loh, and Way [25] with permission.)*

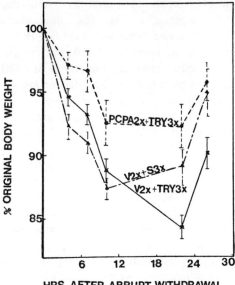

FIG. 6. Tryptophan enhancement of physical dependence and antagonism of the effect by PCPA as indicated by mean body weight loss after abrupt withdrawal. Mice were rendered dependent by pellet implantation for 3 days, and abstinence was induced by removal of the pellet. PCPA 2X denotes PCPA in peanut oil administered 24 hours before and after pellet implantation at a dose of 320 mg/kg, i.p.; V, the peanut oil vehicle; TRY 3X indicates tryptophan, 75 mg/kg, i.p., administered 4 hours before and 20 and 44 hours after implantation. (*From Ho, Loh, and Way* [22], *with permission.*)

the central nervous function dictated the need to assess the effect of the compound on the pharmacology of morphine.

The administration of cAMP intracerebrally in mice prior to morphine antagonized the analgetic effects of the latter compound, as evidenced by the finding that the amount of morphine required to produce analgesia (prolongation of tail-flick reaction time to thermal stimulus) was more than doubled. Surprisingly, cAMP intravenously increased the morphine AD50 as much as cAMP intracerebrally, although a considerably higher dose was required, and the maximum effect was not reached until after 6 hours. Dibutyryl-cAMP, a phosphodiesterase-resistant cAMP analog, and theophylline, a phosphodiesterase inhibitor, also increased the morphine AD50 to a comparable degree. Subjectively, the antagonism of morphine effects by all three compounds appeared to persist for at least 24 hours [23, 26].

The antagonism of morphine analgesia by cAMP appeared to have a relationship with the biogenic amines. The administration of dihydroxy-phenylserine (DOPS) to elevate brain norpinephrine largely antagonized the cAMP-induced increase in the morphine AD50, whereas increasing brain 5-HT with its precursor tryptophan enhanced the effects of cAMP. Increasing brain 5-HT and catecholamines by inhibiting their destruction with the monoamine oxidase inhibitor, pargyline, resulted in antagonism of the cAMP effects. Hence, it would appear that elevating brain catecholamines is more critical than lowering 5-HT for reversing cAMP antagonism of morphine antinociception [23, 26].

The antagonistic effects of cAMP on morphine analgesia were even more evident in morphine-tolerant mice. In animals to be rendered tolerant by pellet implantation, the morphine AD50 was increased fourfold by a daily injection of cAMP for 3 days. In nontolerant animals implanted with a dummy pellet, the antagonism by cAMP was but twofold. Thus, it appeared that cAMP affected not only the response of the tolerant animal to morphine but the development of the tolerance as well. To establish more firmly that cAMP could enhance tolerance development to morphine, we used a single injection of cAMP or saline before morphine pellet implantation in mice. After 3 days allowed for tolerance to develop, the morphine AD50 of the group treated 80 hours earlier with cAMP was found to be markedly increased over that of morphine-implanted mice pretreated with saline (Figure 7). Although an increase in morphine AD50 (decreased analgetic response) was noted to occur after acute administration of cAMP, this effect could be dissociated temporally from that accelerating morphine tolerance development. Thus, the accelerating effect of cAMP on tolerance development appears to be distinct from its antagonist action on morphine antinociception, and possibly different neurohumoral processes are involved with each effect [24].

Enhancement of physical dependence by cAMP was also demonstrated in mice receiving a single injection of cAMP 2 hours before morphine pellet implantation. The amount of naloxone needed to precipitate withdrawal jumping 80 hours later was less than one-third that of the control. Figure 8 further demonstrates acceleration of morphine dependence by cAMP, showing that the weight loss occurring after removal of the implanted pellet from dependent mice can be enhanced two- to threefold by cAMP pretreatment. The accelerated development of both tolerance to and dependence on morphine was blocked by the concurrent injection of cycloheximide [24].

On the basis of the cAMP findings, the interactions of morphine with adrenergic receptor blockers also seemed to merit investigation. Robinson and coworkers [45] had suggested that the alpha and beta adrenergic receptors are regulatory subunits of adenylcyclase. They noted that stimulation of the beta receptor was accompanied by an increase in intracellular adenyl cyclase activity and postulated that the beta receptor is an integral part of the adenyl cyclase system. Chow and his associates [11] found that the acute administration of

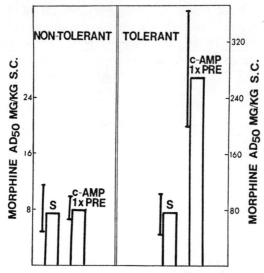

FIG. 7. Enhancement of morphine tolerance development by a single dose of cAMP. Mice were rendered tolerant by morphine pellet implantation for 3 days. A single dose of cAMP(10 mg/kg, i.v.) or saline (S) was administered 2 hours prior to pellet implantation. Non-tolerant mice received a dummy pellet implant. The morphine AD50 and 95% C. L. were determined 6 hours after pellet removal (or 80 hours after cAMP). (*From Ho, Loh, and Way* [24], *with permission.*)

morphine increased significantly brain adenyl cyclase activity in mice both *in vivo* and *in vitro*, and that the activity was reduced after development of tolerance to morphine. Chasin et al. [8] indicated the presence of alpha and beta adrenergic receptors in various brain areas which can be differentiated with appropriate adrenergic blocking agents.

To assess the role of adrenergic blockade on morphine tolerance and physical dependence development the β-blocker, dichloroisoproterenol (DCI), was studied in mice implanted with a pellet of morphine. Administration of DCI for 3 days resulted in the slowing of tolerance development, as evidenced by the comparative effects of the treatment on the ratio of the morphine AD50 in morphine and control animals. In the saline-treated mice implanted with morphine an 11-fold tolerance developed, but in implanted animals treated with DCI only a 4-fold tolerance developed. DCI also slowed the development of dependence. When the DCI was given prior to and during the development of dependence, the naloxone ED50 was 8 times greater than in implanted animals treated with saline [4]. On the other hand, α-blockers failed to inhibit tolerance and dependence development [36].

The precise mechanism by which morphine and exogenous cAMP may interact is still unclear. Any conclusions concerning such action must be tempered by consideration of its widespread effects on many physiologic and biochemic systems. Nonetheless, from a pharmacologic viewpoint, the potency ratio of cAMP for eliciting the response appears to be high. The accelerating effect of cAMP on morphine tolerance and physical dependence was achieved at one-fortieth the dose which produced no fatalities or overt toxic signs [23, 24].

The findings with cAMP appear to have considerable import even though its CNS functions are not fully known. Whatever the mechanism of cAMP action, our data suggest that it may possess long-range effects that have not been

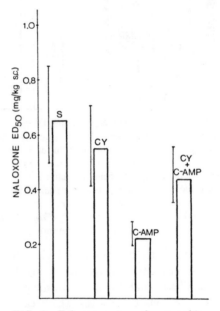

FIG. 8. Enhancement of morphine physical dependence development by cAMP and its inhibition by cycloheximide as measured by the naloxone ED50-precipitated withdrawal jumping. Mice were rendered dependent by morphine pellet implantation for 3 days. CY + cAMP denotes mice receiving daily injections of cycloheximide, i.p., plus a single i.v. injection of cAMP 2 hours before pellet implantation; cAMP, the group receiving the same dose of cAMP plus daily injections of saline, i.p.; CY, the group injected with saline i.v. before implantation plus daily i.p. injections of cycloheximide; S, the group receiving both the i.v. and i.p. injections of saline. (*From Ho, Loh, and Way* [24] , *with permission.*)

realized. It appears highly significant that the compound should accelerate morphine tolerance and dependence development and that a single dose should elicit an effect that is evident after more than 3 days. Since tryptophan, like cAMP, antagonizes morphine antinociception and accelerates the development of tolerance and physical dependence, there may well be a link between the two substances. Consistent with this viewpoint are the findings of Shein and Wurtman [47], who reported that serotonin synthesis in cultured rat pineal gland was stimulated by cAMP; and, recently, Tagliamonte et al. [51] found that dibutyryl cAMP increased the serotonin turnover in rat brain after lateral ventricular administration. The evidence, while only circumstantial, thus provides a heuristic basis for further tests.

The inhibition of the cAMP accelerating effects on morphine tolerance and dependence by cycloheximide suggests that some protein or macromolecule is involved. There is mounting evidence that cAMP may play a role in enzyme induction, at least in the liver [61]. Although a peripheral action of cAMP cannot be excluded, it should not be surprising that with pharmacologic doses some cyclic AMP may gain access to the CNS. Despite the plethora of publications on cAMP, studies *in vivo* on its pharmacologic actions and biologic disposition are rare, and such studies are much needed to provide the answers to our conjectures.

γ-Amino Butyric Acid (GABA)

The possible involvement of GABA in the inhibitory processes of vertebrates as well as of invertebrates has been seriously considered. There is increasing evidence that GABA acts as an inhibitory neurotransmitter at certain brain synapses. In preliminary studies, the compound was found to antagonize morphine antinociception acutely in the mouse; but with repeated administration it also accelerated both morphine tolerance and physical dependence development, as measured in the usual manner in morphine pellet-implanted mice. Similar but more pronounced effects were obtained with amino-oxyacetic acid, which inhibits the transamination of GABA. On the other hand, reverse effects were obtained with bicuculline, an antagonist of GABA. Bicuculline was observed to inhibit both tolerance and dependence development [21].

SUMMARY AND CONCLUSIONS

There are many pharmacologic manipulations that can greatly modify the development of tolerance to and physical dependence on morphine. The rate of development of either syndrome may be reduced or accelerated. Furthermore, the alteration can be achieved with a dose of an agent that may or may not alter morphine responses acutely.

Several compounds, it appears, can inhibit or reduce morphine tolerance and dependence by diverse mechanisms. There are at least five levels of activity where such an action can apparently be mediated by the following drugs or classes of drugs: (*a*) narcotic antagonists such as naloxone, (*b*) inhibitors of protein synthesis, (*c*) inhibitors of serotonin synthesis, (*d*) β-adrenergic blockers, and (*e*) γ-aminobutyric acid antagonists such as bicuculline. Conversely, tolerance and dependence can be accelerated with agents which oppose the effects of the last three classes of compounds. These agents are, respectively: a stimulator of serotonin synthesis (tryptophan), cAMP and its analogs, and inhibitors of GABA transamination.

Evidence has been presented that the processes associated with the development of tolerance to and physical dependence on morphine can be selectively separated from those involved in acute morphine action. On the other hand, the processes involved in the development of tolerance and dependence appear to be intimately associated. Despite various pharmacologic manipulations, which have served to alter the acute effects of morphine and to inhibit or enhance tolerance and physical dependence development, none has resulted unequivocally in dissociating tolerance from dependence development. We interpret this to mean that closely underlying mechanisms in the CNS are involved for both processes. In our studies, we have found it convenient to assess the role of each neurotransmitter separately. However, it should be recognized that morphine could affect several neurohormones whose functions are likely to be intimately enmeshed. Indeed, a critical balance between the substances may be more important than any single transmitter.

The withdrawal signs resulting from morphine abstinence appear to involve norepinephrine, dopamine, and acetylcholine. Although these three substances may participate in the acute and withdrawal responses to morphine, apparently they are not the crucial ones involved directly with tolerance and physical dependence development. On the other hand, 5-HT does seem to be involved with the latter conditions. Its precise role in the two syndromes is unclear, but a relationship is suggested by the fact that reduction of 5-HT synthesis by two agents (PCPA and DHT), acting by diverse mechanisms resulted in an inhibition of tolerance and dependence development. Conversely, stimulation of 5-HT synthesis by precursor (tryptophan) loading effected an enhancement in tolerance and dependence development. Moreover, the acceleration of the two processes by tryptophan could be blocked by PCPA

Evidence has been obtained indicating that the mechanisms involved in tolerance and physical dependence can be dissociated from those more directly related to the acute responses to morphine; such indications, however, do not necessarily mean that these processes are totally unrelated. Indeed, we have some evidence suggesting that they are very likely entwined. Certain compounds (tryptophan, cAMP, GABA) and their surrogates, which antagonize the acute antinociceptive actions of morphine, appear to accelerate tolerance and dependence development. Conversely, their respective antagonists tend to enhance morphine analgesia and appear to delay the development of tolerance and physical dependence.

The findings that the processes involved in the acute responses to morphine can be dissociated selectively from those involved in the development of tolerance to and physical dependence on morphine have important therapeutic implications. Our experimental studies appear to form a basis for possible clinical use of a pharmacologic agent which would prevent the development of narcotic tolerance and physical dependence without modifying analgetic efficacy. For the present, the compounds available for such purposes are much too toxic to be used in human subjects over prolonged periods, but it is likely that safer agents could be designed for such purposes. The testing of such compounds would present difficulties. Ethical questions concerning the feasibility of testing our hypothesis in man would certainly be raised, since it would be necessary to render subjects physically dependent on morphine. But perhaps this objection might be overcome if the subjects were terminal cancer patients who have been prescribed narcotics.

The successful development of such an agent would also have sociolegal implications. If narcotic tolerance and dependence can be prevented without altering analgesia, then it is likely that euphoria also would not be modified. The latter action and drive-reducing effects of morphine in conjunction with psychic elements of the individual may be deemed primarily responsible for promoting compulsive drug use, but there is little question that the development of tolerance and particularly physical dependence strongly reinforce the drive to obtain the drug. It is thus within the realm of possibility that an agent, by preventing the physical facets of heroin dependence, would decrease the need to use heroin repetitively on a continuing basis, with a subsequent reduction of the antisocial activity that generally occurs when the addict is going off drugs.

REFERENCES

1. Algeri, S., & Costa, E. Physical dependence on morphine fails to increase serotonin turnover rate in rat brain. *Biochem. Pharmacol.*, 20, 877, 1971.
2. Azmitia, E. C., Hess, P., & Reis, D. Tryptophan hydroxylase changes in midbrain of rat after chronic morphine administration. *Life Sci.*, 9, 633, 1970.
3. Baumgarten, H. G., Evetts, K. D., Holman, R. B., Iversen, L. L., Vogt, Marthe, & Wilson, Gay. Effects of 5,6-dihydroxytryptamine on monoaminergic neurones in the central nervous system of the rat. *J. Neurochem.*, 19, 1587, 1972.
4. Bhargava, H. N., Chan, S. L., & Way, E. Leong. Effect of β-adrenergic blockage on morphine analgesia, tolerance and physical dependence. *Proceedings of the Western Pharmacol. Soc.*, 15, 4, 1972.
5. Bhargava, H. N., & Way, E. Leong. Acetylcholinesterase inhibition and morphine effects in morphine tolerant and dependent mice. *J. Pharmacol. Exp. Ther.*, 183, 31, 1972.
6. Bloom, F. E., Algeri, S., Groppetti, A., Revuelta, A., & Costa, E. Lesion of central norepinephrine terminals with 6-OH-dopamine: biochemistry and fine structure. *Science*, 166, 1284, 1969.
7. Bowers, M. B., & Kleber, H. D. Methadone increases mouse brain 5-hydroxyindoleacetic acid. *Nature* (London), 229, 134, 1971.

8. Chasin, M., Rivkin, I., Mamrak, F., Samaniego, S. G., & Hess, S. M. α- and β-adrenergic receptors as mediators of accumulation of cyclic adenosine 3',5'-monophosphate in specific areas of guinea pig brain. *J. Biol. Chem.*, 246, 3037, 1971.

9. Cheney, D. L., & Costa, E. Rebuttal to Hitzemann et al. [20]. *Science* (Washington), 178, 646, 1972.

10. Cheney, D. L., Goldstein, A., Algeri, S., & Costa, E. Narcotic tolerance and dependence: lack of relationship with brain serotonin turnover. *Science* (Washington), 171, 1169, 1971.

11. Chou, W. S., Ho, A. K. S., & Loh, H. H. Effect of acute and chronic morphine and norepinephrine on brain adenyl cyclase activity. *Proceedings of the Western Pharmacol. Soc.*, 14, 42, 1971.

12. Clouet, D. H., & Ratner, M. Catecholamine biosynthesis in brains of rats treated with morphine. *Science*, 168, 854, 1970.

13. Collier, H. O. J. A general theory of the genesis of drug dependence by induction of receptors. *Nature* (London), 205, 181, 1965.

14. Fernstrom, J. D., & Wurtman, R. J. Brain serotonin content: physiological dependence on plasma tryptophan levels. *Science*, 173, 149, 1971.

15. Florendo, N. T., Barnett, R. J., & Greengard, P. Cyclic 3',5'-nucleotide phosphodiesterase: cytochemical localization in cerebral cortex. *Science* (Washington), 173, 745, 1971.

16. Friedler, G., Bhargava, H. N., Quock, R., & Way, E. Leong. The effect of 6-hydroxydopamine on morphine tolerance and physical dependence. *J. Pharmacol. Exp. Ther.*, 183, 49, 1972.

17. Gessa, G. L., Krishna, G., Forn, J., Tagliamonte, A., & Brodie, B. B. Behavioral and vegetative effects produced by dibutyryl cyclic AMP injected into different areas of the brain. In P. Greengard & E. Costa (Eds.), *Role of cyclic AMP in cell function.* New York: Raven Press, 1970.

18. Greengard, P., & Costa, E. *Role of cyclic AMP in cell function.* New York: Raven Press, 1970.

19. Haubrich, D. R., & Blake, D. E. Effect of acute and chronic administration of morphine on the metabolism of brain serotonin in rats. *Fed. Proc.*, 28, 793, 1969.

20. Hitzemann, R. J., Ho, I. K., & Loh, H. H. Narcotic tolerance, dependence and serotonin turnover. *Science* (Washington), 178, 645, 1972.

21. Ho, I. K., Loh, H. H., & Way, E. Leong. Unpublished data.

22. Ho, I. K., Loh, H. H., & Way, E. Leong. Influence of 1-tryptophan on morphine analgesia, tolerance and physical dependence. Presented at 34th meeting of the NAS–NRC Committee on Problems of Drug Dependence, Ann Arbor, May 1972.

23. Ho, I. K., Loh, H. H., & Way, E. Leong. Cyclic AMP antagonism of morphine analgesia. *J. Pharmacol. Exp. Ther.*, 185, 336–346, 1973.

24. Ho, I. K., Loh, H. H., & Way, E. Leong. Effects of cyclic AMP on morphine tolerance and physical dependence. *J. Pharmacol. Exp. Ther.*, 185, 347–357, 1973.

25. Ho, I. K., Loh, H. H., & Way, E. Leong. Influence of 5,6-dihydroxytryptamine on morphine tolerance and physical dependence. *Europ. J. Pharmacol.*, 21, 331–336, 1973.

26. Ho, I. K., Lu, S. E., Loh, H. H., & Way, E. L. Effect of cyclic AMP on morphine analgesia, tolerance and physical dependence. *Nature* (London), 238, 397, 1972.

27. Ho, I. K., Lu, S. E., Stolman, S., Loh, H. H., & Way, E. Leong. Influence of p-chlorophenylalanine on morphine tolerance and physical dependence and regional brain serotonin turnover studies in morphine tolerant-dependent mice. *J. Pharmacol. Exp. Ther.*, 182, 155, 1972.

28. Hosoya, E. Some withdrawal symptoms of rats to morphine. *Pharmacologist*, 1, 77, 1959.

29. Huidobro, F., Contreras, E., & Croxatto, R. Studies on morphine III action of metabolic precursors to serotonin and noradrenaline and related substances in the

abstinence syndrome to morphine in white mice. *Arch. Intern. Pharmacodyn.*, **146**, 444, 1963.

30. Huidobro, F., & Maggiolo, C. Some features of the abstinence syndrome to morphine in mice. *Acta Physiol. Latinoamer.*, 18, 201, 1961.
31. Iwamoto, E. T., Ho, I. K., & Way, E. Leong. Sudden elevation of brain dopamine after naloxone-precipitated withdrawal in morphine-dependent mice and rats. Presented at the meeting of the Western Pharmacological Society, January 1973.
32. Knapp, Suzanne, & Mandell, A. J. Parachlorophenylalanine–its three phase sequence of interactions with the two forms of brain tryptophan hydroxylase. *Life Sci.*, 2, 16, 761–771, 1972.
33. Koe, B. K., & Weissman, A. *p*-Chlorophenylalanine: a specific depletor of brain serotonin. *J. Pharmacol. Exp. Ther.*, 154, 499, 1966.
34. Loh, H. H., Cho, T. M., Ho, I. K., & Way, E. Leong. Regulation of brain serotonin biosynthesis in morphine tolerant mice, in preparation.
35. Loh, H. H., Hitzemann, R. J., Craves, F., & Way, E. Leong. The relationship of morphine analgesia to adrenergic mechanisms. Problems of Drug Dependence, National Academy of Science–National Research Council, Vol. 2, 1573–1585, 1971.
36. Loh, H. H., Ho, I. K., & Craves, F. Personal communication.
37. Loh, H. H., Shen, F. H., & Way, E. Leong. Inhibition of morphine tolerance and physical dependence development and brain serotonin synthesis by cycloheximide. *Biochem. Pharmacol.*, 18, 2711, 1969.
38. Mandell, A. J., Segal, D. S., Kucenski, R. T., & Knapp, S. Some factors in the regulation of the brain's neurotransmitter biosynthetic enzymes and receptor sensitivity, drug mechanisms and behavior. In J. McGough (Ed.), *Brain chemistry and behavior*, 1972, in press.
39. Marshall, I., & Grahame-Smith, D. G. Evidence against a role of brain 5-hydroxytryptamine in the development of physical dependence upon morphine in mice. *J. Pharmacol. Exp. Ther.*, 179, 634, 1971.
40. Maruyama, Y., Hayashi, G., Smits, S. E., & Takemori, A. E. Studies on the relationship between 5-hydroxytryptamine turnover in brain and tolerance and physical dependence in mice. *J. Pharmacol. Exp. Ther.*, 178, 20, 1971.
41. McAffee, D. A., Schorderet, M., & Greengard, P. Adenosine $3',5'$-monophosphate in nervous tissue: increase associated with synaptic transmission. *Science* (Washington), 171, 1156, 1971.
42. Miyamoto, E., Kuo, J. F., & Greengard, P. Andnosine $3',5'$-monophosphate dependent protein kinase from brain. *Science*, 165, 63, 1969.
43. Neff, N. H., Tozer, T. N., & Brodie, B. B. Application of steady-state kinetics to studies of the transfer of 5-hydroxyindoleacetic acid from brain to plasma. *J. Pharmacol. Exp. Ther.*, 158, 214, 1967.
44. Porter, C. C., Tataro, J. A., & Stone, C. A. Effect of 6-hydroxydopamine and some other compounds on the concentration of norepinephrine in the hearts of mice. *J. Pharmacol. Exp. Ther.*, 140, 308, 1963.
45. Robinson, G. A., Butcher, R. W., & Sutherland, E. W. Adenyl cyclase as an adrenergic receptor. *Ann. N.Y. Acad. Sci.*, 139, 703, 1967.
46. Schecter, P. J., Lovenberg, W., & Sjoerdsma, A. Dissociation of morphine tolerance and dependence from brain serotonin synthesis rate in mice. *Biochem. Pharmacol.*, 21, 751, 1972.
47. Shein, H. M., & Wurtman, R. J. Cyclic adenosine monophosphate: stimulation of melatonin and serotonin synthesis in cultured rat pineals. *Science*, 166, 519, 1969.
48. Shen, F. H., Loh, H. H., & Way, E. Leong. Brain serotonin turnover in morphine tolerant-dependent mice. *J. Pharmacol. Exp. Ther.*, 175, 427, 1970.
49. Shuster, L., Hannam, R. V., & Boyle, W. E., Jr. A simple method for producing tolerance to dihydromorphinone in mice. *J. Pharmacol. Exp. Ther.*, 140, 149, 1963.

50. Smith, C. B., Villareal, J. E., Bednarezyk, H. J., & Sheldon, M. I. Tolerance to morphine-induced increases in (^{14}C) catecholamine synthesis in mouse brain. *Science,* 170, 1106, 1970.
51. Tagliamonte, A., Tagliamonte, P., Forn, J., Perez-Cruet, J., Krishna, G., & Gessa, G. L. Stimulation of brain serotonin synthesis by dibutyryl-cyclic AMP in rats. *J. Neurochem.,* 18, 1191, 1971.
52. Thoenen, H., & Tranzer, J. P. Chemical sympathectomy by selective destruction of adrenergic nerve endings with 6-hydroxydopamine. *Naunyn-Schmiedebergs Arch. Pharmakol,* 261, 557, 1969.
53. Tozer, T. N., Neff, N. H., & Brodie, B. B. Application of steady state kinetics to the synthesis rate and turnover time of serotonin in the brain of normal and reserpine treated rats. *J. Pharmacol. Exp. Ther.,* 153, 177, 1966.
54. Uretsky, N. J., & Iversen, L. L. Effect of 6-hydroxydopamine on catecholamine containing neurons in the rat brain. *J. Neurochem.,* 17, 269, 1970.
55. Way, E. Leong. Brain neurohormones in morphine tolerance and dependence. Fifth Int'l. Cong. of Pharmacol., Vol. 1, pp. 199–216, 1972.
56. Way, E. Leong. Role of serotonin in morphine effects. *Fed. Proc.,* 31, 113, 1972.
57. Way, E. Leong, Loh, H. H., & Shen, F. H. Morphine tolerance, physical dependence and synthesis of brain 5-hydroxytryptamine. *Science* (Washington), 162, 1290, 1968.
58. Way, E. Leong, Loh, H. H., & Shen, F. H. Simultaneous quantitative assessment of morphine tolerance and physical dependence. *J. Pharmacol. Exp. Ther.,* 167, 1, 1969.
59. Way, E. Leong, & Shen, F. H. Catecholamines and 5-hydroxytryptamine. In D. H. Clouet (Ed.), *Narcotic drugs: Biochemical pharmacology.* New York: Plenum Press, 1971.
60. Wei, Eddie, Loh, H. H., & Way, E. Leong. Assessment of precipitated abstinence in morphine dependent rats. *J. Pharmacol. Exp. Ther.,* 184, 398, 1973.
61. Wicks, W. D. Regulation of hepatic enzyme synthesis by cyclic AMP. *Ann. N.Y. Acad. Sci.,* 185, 152, 1971.

PART II CLINICAL APPROACHES TO THE TREATMENT AND CONTROL OF OPIATE ADDICTION

SECTION 1
INTRODUCTION

Joel Elkes
Johns Hopkins University School of Medicine

Our College has always conducted a conversation between the *somatic* and the *symbolic*; to which we now add the dusty, dirty problem of the street. It would be nice if revolutions came one at a time. But revolutions do not oblige, and come in battalions; and their symptoms—the national fevers and obsessions—crowd in hard, one upon the other. We have been hit hard in the sixties: the murders, the riots, the war, sex, dress, hair, hoopla, and holiness. We have come from "there" to "here." And, in looking forward, in 1972, we are still left with the broad phenomena of youth, of family, of the school—which, in our professional jargon, we continue to call "adolescent disorders," "juvenile delinquency," and "drug abuse." Some profound questions have been raised by these phenomena; questions about where, who, and what neuropsychopharmacologists are as a profession; what business we have doing what we are doing; or, for that matter, what our business really is.

We rightly question the validity of our methods, the usefulness of our evaluations. Above all, do our methods work? As always, fear is a great propellant, and marshals unexpected resources; and when fear is coupled with incentive—grant incentive—things begin to happen. From the illusory safety of our professional turf we recognize the dimensions, the depth, the cultural and historical embeddedness of the problem of addiction—to drugs, to alcohol, to tobacco—to the prescriptions drugs, dispensed or self-dispensed.

The basic economics of supply and demand stand out as powerful factors: the streamlined business organization of the heroin traffic; the eloquent fiscal returns of the tobacco and alcohol industries; the production figures for some common drugs, like amphetamines and barbiturates—far, far in excess of therapeutic need, clearly making their way into the illicit market. Is supply

123

and crass material gain in a predatory drug culture an operant? Clearly it is. Is social contact and social reinforcement a vector of spread, making drug addiction, in the true public health sense, a communicable disorder? It looks that way. Do the media and misguided, haranguing, educational programs inflate the problems, and exercise a multiplier effect? It looks that way. Could they conversely be used to relieve, and to involve people in their own decision making? Very probably, yes. Do the models given by parents enhance both susceptibility and resistance? Very likely. Is the family fading as a school of social learning? Definitely, yes. Can schools and, especially, peers do more? Again, the evidence is positive. As the saying goes, "more research is needed"—research of a kind of *applied* scholarship, which cuts through the strident tones of a field in crisis, giving way to a sense of order and understanding, which indeed is the business of our College: understanding of the full social context of the problem; of the many areas which compound it, and which must be articulated and connected to yield both a view and a solution. Understanding, above all, of the historical process, and the truly huge shift in values in our fragile society which these changes portend.

In this process, we must clearly distinguish what is medicine's and what is not; what belongs to the law and the law's enforcement; what to education, to the home and the community; and, above all, what is the basis upon which sensible public policy can be built. As physicians, pharmacologists, and behavioral scientists, we have our place, to be sure. But when it comes to deep-seated social problems which we face, we are mere witnesses, and our functions are remedial.

When people die in slums, they die not only of overdose, but sometimes of undetected murder. Housing, hygiene, nutrition, and neglect is the business of everybody. We had better be careful to accept the limits of our responsibilities, and to toss any hot potato that is thrown our way straight back where it came from.

Now, it is a feature of the field of opiate addiction that, like no other, it compels an articulation of concepts, services and resources, and attitudes, which conceivably could serve as a model in many other areas of health service and mental health care. The shift in the drug addiction field from law enforcement to medicine is significant; the shift from medicine to far-reaching social legislation is inevitable.

For these reasons, the creation by the White House and Congress, in June of 1971, of the Special Action Office for Drug Abuse Prevention is a historic step. In bringing together and collating the work of some 18 agencies, this office has, despite formidable obstacles, already greatly enhanced the collective yield of respective resources. It has blasted holes into some bureaucratic walls, and started identifying and counting cases on a nationwide basis, making it possible to get an idea of the characteristics and natural course of the epidemic and the effectiveness of countermeasures. Taking a public health approach, it has asked some hard questions, at the core of which is: Which procedures work, and which do not? At the head of this office is Dr. Jerome Jaffe, a member of our College of long standing, who, in his own state of Illinois some years ago, conceived, planned, and executed a remarkable program in which a multimodality approach was tied to evaluation of effectiveness. It is still regarded as a model by many states (including my own, of Maryland). Following Dr. Jaffe's paper, Dr. Thomas Bewley, director of three important drug abuse programs in London, discusses the differences between the British approach and our own: differences stemming from differences in numbers, in attitudes, and the respective cultures. Finally, Dr. Matthew Dumont, Assistant Commissioner for Drug Rehabilitation in the State of Massachusetts, focuses on another key problem: Is the drug addict the carrier and vessel of society's fears?

MULTIMODALITY APPROACHES TO THE TREATMENT AND PREVENTION OF OPIATE ADDICTION

Jerome H. Jaffe
Special Action Office for Drug Abuse Prevention
Executive Office of the President

Presentations by an administrator before scientific audiences inevitably raise two questions. First, is there a relationship between the administrator's own previous scientific activity and present policies? Second, to what extent does a scientific presentation contain or represent policy in the making? I have found no easy answers to these questions. But knowing that the questions are inevitably raised, I have taken two steps to clarify the situation. First, I have based this presentation largely on a paper presented at a symposium of the American Federation of Clinical Research in May, 1971, preceding any discussions of my present administrative responsibilities. Second, where I do interject some views on policy, I have tried to label them clearly as such.

This presentation differs from the one given 18 months ago in two respects. First, I would like to add some thoughts about patterns of opiate use that precede the development of compulsive use. Second, I would like to acknowledge that compulsive opiate use not associated with excessive consumption of other psychoactive drugs (such as barbiturates, alcohol, amphetamines) is rapidly joining the American bison as a species that, although not extinct, is now rarely seen.

It remains true now, as it has for untold generations, that the less effective our treatment methods for any given syndrome, the wider the diversity of opinions on how best to approach it. So it is with the syndrome of compulsive narcotics use, and so it is with our approaches to the prevention of this syndrome. With respect to treatment, several conceptually distinct approaches are still in operation. They differ not only in the ways in which narcotics users are handled, but also in the premises upon which the treatment operations are based, and in the goals that they are trying to reach. To compare these approaches with respect to effectiveness, it is not necessary that they be based on similar views of etiology or proceed from identical premises. It does seem axiomatic, however, that comparisons of these approaches to each other will be meaningful only if they are trying to reach the same goals. However, there is still no agreement on what goals should be given priority. There is a general consensus that, ideally, all compulsive narcotics users would become law-abiding, productive, non-drug-using, emotionally stable, independent members of the community, but disagreement breaks out over which goal will be given emphasis if it becomes apparent that all elements in the ideal set of goals cannot be reached. It is becoming clearer that these goals are not inextricably intertwined, and that different patterns of outcome for different types of patients participating in different treatment programs are the rule and not the exception.

There are at least eight conceptually and operationally distinct treatment approaches to the compulsive opioid use syndrome. Realizing that in naming and describing we often betray our biases, I have nevertheless decided to continue to use the same designations that I used almost two years ago. These approaches, or models, are as follows:

1. Medical-distributive
2. Supervisory-deterrent
3. Self-regulating community (character restructuring)
4. Psychotherapeutic
5. Benign maintenance/specific defect correction
6. Conditioning-narcotics antagonist
7. Faith and dedication
8. Multimodality

I will elaborate on each of the individual models only briefly.

The *medical-distributive* model in its simplest terms is based on the premise that compulsive narcotics use is a syndrome poorly understood, but probably due to multiple causes. A companion premise is that the syndrome is virtually impossible to treat and that society and the individual are best served when that individual is given access to the narcotic drugs he wishes to use under medical supervision. This is essentially the system now employed in England, where specialized clinics are set up to supervise the prescribing of heroin to heroin users.

However, since narcotics are provided for intravenous self-administration, the complications of intravenous use are present. Furthermore, since patients are given quantities of heroin for self-administration at home, there is no way to prevent illicit diversion.

Related to the medical-distributive model, but conceptually quite different from it, is what I have chosen to call the *benign maintenance/specific defect correction* model. Actually, these are two separable models that I have condensed for convenience of presentation because, in practice, they involve the same clinical operations over the first 6 to 18 months of treatment. In this model, compulsive narcotics use is recognized as a chronic relapsing syndrome, and any medicine that can permit an individual to become a productive citizen is viewed as an appropriate therapeutic agent. The proponents of the specific defect model view the repeated return to narcotics as a manifestation of a specific "narcotics hunger" that is, in turn, due to metabolic changes produced by chronic use of high doses of narcotics. The benign-maintenance proponents do not necessarily accept this view of a specific narcotics-induced defect and believe that patients can be successfully withdrawn after social stabilization has been achieved. The supporters of either model agree that a significant number of compulsive heroin users can become reasonably productive citizens when provided with regular doses of oral methadone or other substances.

These approaches differ from the medical-distributive model in the pains taken to ensure that the drug is used only in oral form. The objective is not to provide a legalized euphoria, which is precisely what the medical-distributive model does provide.

The *supervisory-deterrent* model is based on the premise that whatever underlying social, biochemical, or psychological factors may make one person more susceptible to narcotics use than another, the individual who is not physically dependent can still choose, in large degree, whether or not to use a narcotic. The fundamental operation in this model is withdrawal from narcotics use, usually in an institutional setting, followed by supervision in the community. If there is evidence of a return to narcotics use, the individual may be required to return to the institutional setting for an additional period. This general approach has been used by both medically oriented and correctional systems; it is the primary premise on which civil commitment and parole programs are operated.

In the *character-restructuring, self-regulating therapeutic community*, drug use is viewed as a manifestation of immaturity and an incapacity to delay gratification. To correct this, the patient is required to undergo maturation and character change during a period of 12 to 18 months' residence in a community largely run by ex-addicts. In general, all these programs tend to be highly selective in admitting patients to treatment. Prospective residents must demonstrate their motivation by expressing, among other things, a willingness to undergo abrupt withdrawal from narcotics. The drop-out rate is high. The individual who remains for a year or more appears to undergo significant changes in his outlook on life, but adequate follow-up studies on the adjustment of those who successfully complete treatment are still lacking.

The *conditioning-antagonist* model is based on the hypothesis that, in addition to any characterological problems that may have antedated narcotics use, individuals who become narcotics users acquire a complex set of instrumentally and classically conditioned reflexes. Thus, each injection of an opiate, by producing a positive reinforcement or alleviating distress, increases the tendency to make a similar drug-using response. With repeated use, physical dependence develops. The withdrawal syndrome produces a regularly recurring distress, increasing the occasions for reinforcing drug-using behavior. Further-more, withdrawal symptoms may become conditioned to the environment, so that long after withdrawal is completed a return to the environment in which drug use occurred elicits conditioned withdrawal phenomena to which the former narcotics user responds by re-initiating the drug-use cycle.

Theoretically, to extinguish such behavior the narcotics user should be permitted to engage in drug-using behavior but get no reinforcement. Theoreti-cally, such a situation can be brought about by administering a narcotic antagonist on a chronic basis. If the drug user elects to use a narcotic he will feel no narcotic effect. Furthermore, even regular use will not lead to physical dependence, and to a considerable degree the likelihood of an overdose is reduced. Dr. Wikler has presented the experimental evidence for these hypotheses elsewhere in this book.

The *psychotherapeutic* model is based on the premise that drug dependence is a manifestation of problems that antedate drug use, that many of these problems are psychological or interpersonal, and that relapse after withdrawal is likely to occur unless these problems are resolved. Proponents of this view generally arrange to withdraw the patient from drugs, usually in a hospital setting, and then continue to provide treatment after the individual returns to the community. During the period of withdrawal, and for some time thereafter, the patient participates in individual or group therapy aimed at ameliorating the problems that led to and perpetuate the drug addiction problem.

Faith and dedication is an approach that should not be overlooked even though it cannot be developed at will. Apparently, for many drug users, the drug-using behavior is based as much on the way it structures life and gives it meaning as it is on the pharmacological effects of the substance being used. From time to time such individuals find other values more meaningful than those of the drug-using subculture. Whether these be turning to religious beliefs of other lands, returning to the religion of their forefathers, or dedicating themselves to secular political activity, the behavioral changes can be rapid and profound.

Multimodality is a term which was originally coined to describe a very specific form of program. At first, it was not meant to convey merely an eclectic view or to acknowledge the selective value of a range of models. It was intended to describe a situation in which a number of very distinct treatment approaches were synthesized under a single administrative structure. The concept has evolved in the last several years. At first, the rivalry between models was such that a program could call itself "multimodality" if proponents of various models (e.g., benign maintenance, traditional psychotherapeutic, self-regulating com-munity) were within a single administrative structure and were willing to sit down for civil discussions. For a brief period it did in fact come to describe a treatment facility within which a wide range of treatment modalities should be offered (e.g., short- or long-term residence in a self-regulating community while abstinent or while maintained on methadone, outpatient methadone maintenance, abstinence and group psychotherapy, or the use of antagonists). More recently, it has come to mean only an eclecticism that perhaps is a realistic response to a difficult problem. Under such an eclectic view (described in this book by Dr. Alfred Freedman), while all the models may be held applicable, different factors may weigh more heavily with one patient than with another, and different approaches may be needed for the same patient at different stages of his or her life. The use of the concept has now become so broad that it is possible to have methadone programs that offer only methadone maintenance but "believe in" a "multimodality" approach. The belief is demonstrated by the existence of working relationships with administratively distinct programs using nonmaintenance approaches. Conversely, some of the latter programs adamantly refuse to use methadone themselves, but believe it might be helpful for some patients and are willing to refer patients to programs that do use it.

Having defined these various models in their pure form and redefined multimodality as a synonym for the eclectic view, I would like to discuss how the limits of this set of responses have shaped policies in the areas of treatment, research, and prevention, not only at the Federal level, but also in many cases at the state and local level.

Stated in the most general terms, a major goal of the efforts of the Federal Government in this area has been to reduce opiate addiction and/or its social cost. We recognize that social cost is itself a composite that includes the cost of the medical and social problems of the user, crimes related to drug use, and the cost of the treatment and law enforcement efforts.

A survey of opiate addiction in the United States in mid-1971 brought some obvious features to the fore. One was that many people who wanted treatment could not get it. We believe that, even though the relative effectiveness of these various approaches had not yet been clearly defined, it was an appropriate policy to make available those treatment approaches that we did have to those who wanted them. When we examined the range of alternatives and measured them against the variety of addicts who might seek treatment, the limits of our capacity to respond became clear. With respect to the supervisory-deterrent approach we did not feel that in its pure form, at least, it should be given priority at a time when so many people were actively seeking treatment but could not get it.

We also realized that no matter how effective faith and dedication might be for some, the government could not provide direct financial support for religious or political groups. Moreover, we recognized that whatever the theoretical merit of the conditioning-antagonist model, the pharmacological agents that would permit us to test it operationally and test it fairly were not available.

We recognized the limitations of the maintenance approaches as well as of the self-regulating (therapeutic) communities in responding to those who are not defined as chronic relapsing opiate users. This limitation does not apply, theoretically, at least, to the use of antagonists in preventing the progression of experimentation to compulsive use; the potential utility of narcotics antagonists in prevention programs has led to an intense effort to develop long-acting orally effective antagonists with few or no side effects. (Dr. William Bunney has described this effort elsewhere in this book.)

Given these limitations, we should recognize that up to the present only three major approaches could be expanded by governmental efforts in any substantial way: maintenance with methadone, residence in self-regulating communities (or their day-care equivalents), and the traditional technique of supervised withdrawal from opiates followed by various forms of aftercare (the psychotherapeutic model).

Even with these limitations, the effort of the Federal Government to make treatment available has been large when measured against previous efforts in this field.

The number of directly funded Federal treatment programs has increased from 16 in January 1969, and 24 in January 1970, to almost 400 in December 1972 (Figure 1). Not unexpectedly, the Federal budget reflects this growth. In 1969, the total amount available for treatment and rehabilitation programs was $46 million, while in fiscal year 1973 the total will approach $300 million. This area thus constitutes the largest single category in the Federal drug abuse budget (Figure 2). Law enforcement efforts have also increased, but treatment and rehabilitation continue to represent approximately one-third of the total effort.

Now, what has been the nature of this growth and what policies guided this growth? First, each of the three major approaches has undergone significant expansion. Given the uncertain efficacy of the self-regulating community and the psychotherapeutic models for a wide range of chronic users, and the reports that some individuals who repeatedly relapse in such situations do adjust well on maintenance programs, we concluded that maintenance should at least be available to those who are clearly addicted and could benefit from it. We felt that every community should have a range of options to offer to narcotics users.

A policy that permitted expansion of maintenance programs raised problems of regulation. We consider it essential to prevent the use of maintenance for individuals not already addicted, and to prevent neo-addiction to methadone and overdose deaths from its illicit diversion.

Simple mathematics reveals that at an average dose of 80 mg/day the treatment of 80,000 individuals involves dispensing about 2.5 tons of methadone each year. Even if a small fraction is diverted, the hazard is considerable. Recognizing this hazard, we have been attempting to devise a better system to prevent diversion, and also to develop maintenance drugs that would be long-acting enough to obviate the need to provide medication that can be taken from the clinic. (Dr. Edward Senay (this volume) describes some clinical experiences with one such drug, acetylmethadol.)

The effort to develop guidelines that are responsive to the needs of clinicians and simultaneously clear enough to minimize diversion and provide for a high standard of care has been a long and arduous one. It has consumed more than a year's time, with input and consultations involving hundreds of interested individuals across the country. These regulations, scheduled for publication in mid-December, 1972, become fully effective within 90 days and will be periodically reviewed thereafter.

In spite of the current popularity of maintenance approaches, most experts recognize that opioid maintenance is now associated with excessive use of non-opioids, suggesting that even maintenance programs would require ancillary services such as residential facilities and backup by medical facilities.

It has been our policy over the last 18 months to emphasize that the effort to make maintenance programs available should not obscure the need to expand other approaches. It has been our policy to support the expansion of the residential model and of linking that model to other approaches. The success of that policy can be judged from the following data. In October of 1971, directly funded Federal programs were treating a total of 20,000 patients. Of these, approximately 10,000 were in maintenance programs and 10,000 were in nonmaintenance programs. By September of 1972 the total patient load of directly funded programs had increased to almost 55,000. Of these, approximately 20,000 were in maintenance programs—an increase of 100%, but 34,600 were in nonmaintenance programs—an increase of 240% (Figure 3).

Similarly, we can look at the number of patients in inpatient, residential, and outpatient settings. In October of 1971 these figures were 2,229; 1,561; and 16,818 respectively. By September of 1972 inpatient capacity had increased to 2,614; but the major expansions were in residential and outpatient categories that increased to 4,682 and 47,427 respectively (Figure 4).

I would like to draw attention to the words *directly funded* in the description of Federal programs. This term is used to describe programs receiving support over which a Federal agency exerts some degree of policy control. In addition, many programs are supported by the Federal Government through block grants, revenue sharing arrangements, and third-party payment arrangements (e.g., Medicaid). In these situations, the quality and direction of the programs are determined at the local level. Our analysis of the total client load and kinds of operating programs is, therefore, based entirely on those that are directly funded.

In one area, however, we made a special effort to examine even those programs that were not directly funded. When the Special Action Office was first created, some observers were worried that the Federal Government would overemphasize a narrow methadone maintenance approach and thus decrease interest in efforts to improve nonmaintenance approaches. In that context it is interesting to examine some changes that have occurred in the past six months in all programs that hold IND permits to use the methadone maintenance approach. These were not exclusively maintenance programs, but were programs authorized to use maintenance along with other approaches; only one-third of these programs were receiving their primary support from the Federal Government.

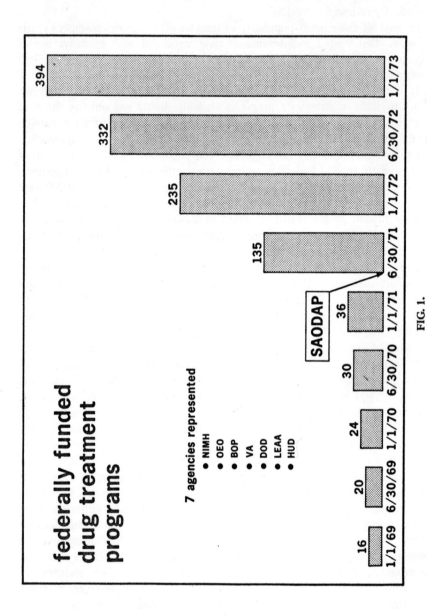

federally funded drug treatment programs

7 agencies represented
- NIMH
- OEO
- BOP
- VA
- DOD
- LEAA
- HUD

SAODAP

16 — 1/1/69
20 — 6/30/69
24 — 1/1/70
30 — 6/30/70
36 — 1/1/71
135 — 6/30/71
235 — 1/1/72
332 — 6/30/72
394 — 1/1/73

FIG. 1.

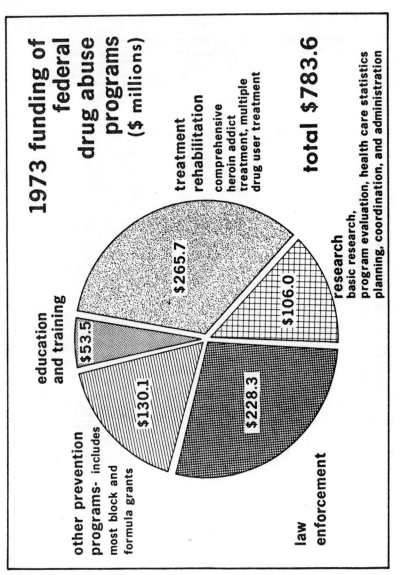

1973 funding of federal drug abuse programs ($ millions)

other prevention programs- includes most block and formula grants

education and training

$53.5

$130.1

$265.7

$228.3

$106.0

treatment rehabilitation

comprehensive heroin addict treatment, multiple drug user treatment

law enforcement

research

basic research, program evaluation, health care statistics planning, coordination, and administration

total $783.6

FIG. 2.

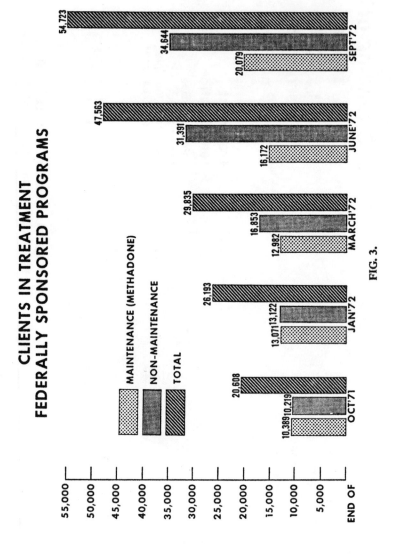

CLIENTS IN TREATMENT
FEDERALLY SPONSORED PROGRAMS

MAINTENANCE (METHADONE)

NON-MAINTENANCE

TOTAL

END OF

55,000
50,000
45,000
40,000
35,000
30,000
25,000
20,000
15,000
10,000
5,000

OCT'71
20,608
10,389 10,219

JAN'72
26,193
13,071 13,122

MARCH'72
29,835
16,853
12,982

JUNE'72
47,563
31,391
16,172

SEPT'72
54,723
34,644
20,079

FIG. 3.

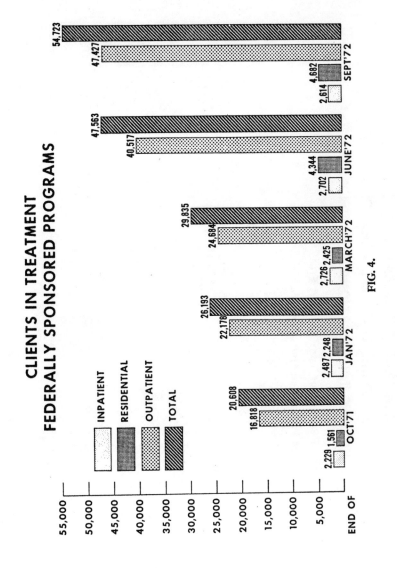

CLIENTS IN TREATMENT
FEDERALLY SPONSORED PROGRAMS

FIG. 4.

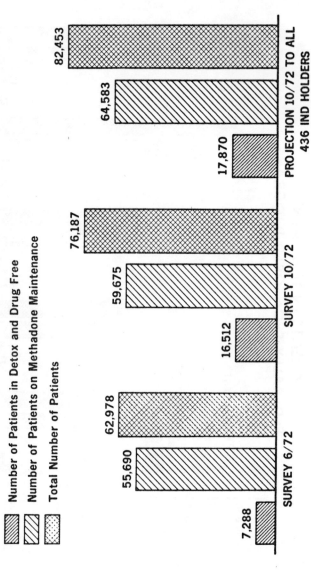

TREATMENT & REHABILITATION CAPACITY
413 LOCAL, STATE, & FEDERAL PROGRAMS
HOLDING INVESTIGATIONAL NEW DRUG PERMITS*

Number of Patients in Detox and Drug Free
Number of Patients on Methadone Maintenance
Total Number of Patients

SURVEY 6/72

7,288
55,690
62,978
16,512

SURVEY 10/72

59,675
76,187
17,870

PROJECTION 10/72 TO ALL
436 IND HOLDERS

64,583
82,453

*Does not include drug free programs which do not hold IND methadone permits

FIG. 5.

These programs were visited by joint teams of FDA and NIMH in the spring of 1972. They were then treating 63,000 people, with 55,700 in maintenance treatment and 7,000 in drug-free or detoxification programs. A telephone survey in September and October of 1972 reached 92% of these programs. Projecting from the 92% to the total group, we found that the following changes had occurred. The total in treatment had increased by 30% to 82,000. However, the group on maintenance had gone up to 64,500, an increase of only 16%, while the drug-free and detoxification groups moved up to almost 18,000, an increase of 150% in about six months (Figure 5).

My inference is that either more and more program directors are adopting the view that patients who have been maintained on methadone can be withdrawn, and that at least an effort in that direction should be made or programs that were once exclusively oriented to maintenance are now developing nonmaintenance components.

I think this is a healthy trend. All the data I have seen over the past year have reinforced my previous view that there is a heterogeneous population of narcotics addicts whose treatment will require diverse approaches.

Space does not permit me to elaborate greatly on prevention. We are interested in developing a situation where the conditioning and biochemical approaches can be given a fair trial. In evolving research priorities in the pharmacological area we have given a high priority to efforts to develop agents that would permit such a trial to occur. I am equally impressed with the possibilities that stem from our increasing understanding of the mechanism of spread among peer groups.

Characteristically, in the major approaches presented here, some action on the part of the drug user or his family initiates the sequence of events that brings him into treatment. Unfortunately, entry into treatment often comes at a stage where drug-using patterns are well established. Hughes and his coworkers at the University of Chicago have been experimenting with techniques that do not wait until this late stage, but link intervention systems to an understanding of the dynamics of the spread of addiction and actively attempt to bring patients into treatment before this occurs.

Yet, we must recognize that our knowledge of the natural history of opiate addiction is far from complete. We cannot be certain how many experimenters would actually become addicted under varying circumstances of peer pressures and availability. Recently Lee Robins and her colleagues completed a follow-up study of Army enlisted men who left Vietnam in September 1971. This study, conducted on behalf of several Federal agencies, found that among men who began heroin use outside the United States, the continued use of heroin after return to their home communities was the exception rather than the rule; and even for those who were dependent on heroin in Vietnam, re-addiction one year after return was still the exception, not the rule.

It is not clear at this point whether the approaches that must be developed for early intervention efforts will fit into any of the eight major categories or combinations thereof presented here. Thus far, however, I have not touched upon what many consider the central issue in this area. Just where does the effort to treat the narcotics user fit into an overall response to this very perplexing problem?

First, I should point out that we have tried to avoid promising more than we can deliver. We recognize that even making all forms of treatment widely available will not ensure that drug users will avail themselves of treatment or that treatment will have any positive effects on the drug users or the communities in which they live. Indeed, we know that even under the best of circumstances many patients show few behavioral changes—narcotics use continues, or, alternatively, new and equally destructive drug use patterns emerge, crime patterns do not always change, and productive activity does not necessarily flow from intensive efforts to provide skills and place people in jobs. Certainly the treatment of the confirmed addict, in and of itself, can have only a limited effect on the patterns of spread that are related to the relatively new drug users.

Having acknowledged these limitations, here and elsewhere, we then confront the realities of our position. What are our alternatives? We do not believe it would be helpful to make all drugs readily available to all citizens; we, therefore, oppose schemes to distribute heroin through medical channels. While there might be some reduction in crime, the other social costs would be unacceptably high. We recognize the limitations of all our present approaches. We hope through a process of careful evaluation to continue to determine which programs are demonstrably effective. Through our efforts to develop mechanisms at the state level we hope to give local groups more responsibility in deciding how to allocate resources to achieve the goals which they feel are most significant.

We recognize that the process of evaluation may be painful, and that we may emerge from it with even more modest claims about our ability to produce positive behavioral change than those which we now make in the optimism of relative ignorance. In the meantime, we hope to make available that which can be offered.

There are many who find it easy to criticize as long as they are not required to offer constructive alternatives. Iconoclastic rhetoric has always been easier to generate than demonstrably effective proposals. We recognize that our present efforts will not solve all problems; however, we believe that the balanced approach we are developing will reduce the social cost of compulsive opiate use, and we will continue to develop this multifaceted approach until more effective alternatives are proposed.

TREATMENT OF OPIATE ADDICTION IN GREAT BRITAIN

Thomas H. Bewley[1]
St. George's, St. Thomas', Tooting Bec Hospitals, England

Past

There have been marked changes in the pattern of opiate dependence in England in the last 20 years. For many years before 1950 the number of people known to be dependent on narcotic drugs was relatively stable, varying between 400 and 600. Those involved tended to be middle-aged and to be disproportionately from the medical and paramedical professions. In most cases, addiction had had a therapeutic origin and the drug involved was usually morphine. Almost coincidental with publication of the first report of an Interdepartmental Committee on Drug Addiction [11] (the first "Brain" Committee report), there originated a series of changes which have continued up to the present. Misuse of illicitly obtained drugs originally appeared in London, but later the problem spread to other parts of the country [15].

The most striking increase was in the number of known young opiate addicts. The majority of these were dependent on heroin, commonly injected intravenously with either cocaine or methylamphetamine. The new cases were nontherapeutic addicts, chiefly in the 18-to-25-year group. The ratio of men to women was 4 to 1. In 1965 the Interdepartmental Committee (the second "Brain" Committee), which had been recalled, recommended certain changes to deal with this [12]. Legislation in the Dangerous Drugs Act 1967 was

[1] I would like to thank the Drugs Branch of the Home Office, particularly Mr. C. G. Jeffery and Mr. H. B. Spear; also Dr. E. R. Bransby of the Department of Health and Social Security; Mr. Thomas Mahon, now at the London School of Economics; and finally Dr. H. H. Blumberg, Dr. D. V. Hawks, and their colleagues at the Addiction Research Unit. This paper consists very largely of a review of the work of all these, to whom I am very grateful.

141

implemented in April 1968 [6]. Notification of addiction to drugs controlled under the Dangerous Drugs Act became compulsory, and the prescribing of heroin or cocaine to an addict could only be carried out by a doctor officially licensed. At the same time the Department of Health and Social Security set up a number of special clinics (the majority in the London area) to treat heroin addicts. In general, only doctors working at these clinics were licensed to prescribe the controlled drugs. Addiction to heroin was still considered an illness, and it continued to be official policy to supply drugs to addicts to maintain their addiction.

Until recently, the figures on which these observations were based were never comprehensive. Before the 1968 legislation it was not obligatory for doctors to report treating drug-dependent patients, and the figures published by the Home Office were largely derived from the routine examination of pharmacists' records. The annual statistics published by the Home Office until 1968 showed only addicts known to have been taking drugs during the previous year. They excluded those not known to be currently taking drugs—for example, addicts who were in prison or abroad or who obtained their drugs entirely from illicit sources [10].

Significant events affecting incidence.   In 1969, Spear attempted to analyze the events of the 1950s which heralded the present situation [15]. He observed that the first significant changes occurred after World War II. A major case of drug trafficking had occurred when approximately 1,200 grains of morphine, mostly in tablet form, and 14 ounces of cocaine were stolen from a firm of wholesale chemists. Although the drugs had been stolen by one of the firm's employees, it transpired that the instigator of the theft was a person having contacts with drug addicts in the West End of London. However, the persons to whom he supplied drugs were already known addicts and there was no evidence that others were recruited to the habit by his activities. A further major case of trafficking occurred in 1951 when the dispensary of a hospital on the borders of London was broken into and considerable quantities of morphine, heroin, and cocaine were stolen. The person involved turned out to be a former employee of the hospital. Although the full extent of his activities cannot be charted, it appears that a majority of those to whom he supplied drugs had no previous experience of heroin addiction. All those ascertained to have received their initial supplies from this source subsequently came to the notice of the Home Office as heroin addicts.

The "British system".   For many years it was believed that there was a formal "British system" whereby opiate addicts could have opiates prescribed for them, and that this somehow led to the very small number of people dependent on drugs in Britain. In fact, there was no system, but as there was very little misuse of drugs this did not matter [2]. Original guidelines for prescribing of opiates to opiate addicts had been laid down in 1926 in a Departmental Committee Report [14]. Addicts for whom morphine or heroin could be prescribed included

Persons for whom, after every effort has been made for the cure of addiction, the drug cannot be completely withdrawn, either because:

(1) complete withdrawal produces serious symptons which cannot be satisfactorily treated under the ordinary condition of private (general) practice; or

(2) the patient, while capable of leading a useful and fairly normal life so long as he takes a certain nonprogressive quantity, usually small, of the drug of addiction, ceases to be able to do so when the regular allowance is withdrawn.

It was also recommended that this course of treatment should not be embarked on without the opinion of a second doctor.

In practice, from the early 1950s, a few doctors were prepared to prescribe heroin for heroin addicts. It was found that when more than was used by an individual was prescribed for him he could, and often did, give, lend, or sell his surplus drugs to other people who could thus become addicted. Irresponsible prescribing in private practice was blamed, and it was decided to transfer the responsibility for prescribing to the Health Service. Thus it came about that special clinics were set up with the aim of prescribing opiates for addicts, although there was no evidence at the time that such treatment was necessarily sound.

Treatment clinics. After the implementation in April 1968 of the 1967 Dangerous Drugs Acts a large number of patients appeared at the new clinics. The majority of doctors working there were swamped, and all they could do at the time was to find out what had been previously prescribed for the individual and continue to prescribe this. Gradually histories were obtained, a better assessment was made of individual patients, and generally the amounts prescribed were reduced [3]. Later it was possible to act in a more rational manner: it became possible to determine whether new patients who attended were using drugs or not, and whether they were physically dependent. At this time, through regular meetings of the doctors working in various clinics, a general system of control was introduced whereby all patients for whom drugs were being prescribed attended at least once weekly and were given prescriptions which could be collected daily. The prescriptions, which were sent to individual chemists, were made out in such a way that the patient could only get one day's supply of drugs at a time on Mondays through Fridays and two days' supply on Saturdays. This has remained the system up to the present. At most of the treatment clinics, routine urine testing for the presence of drugs is done weekly on all patients; it has been found that, although 95% of patients use the drugs that are prescribed for them, 40% use others as well [1].

The workings of the treatment clinics have been reviewed by Gardner and Connell [7, 8], Glatt [9], and Bewley [1, 2, 3], and Stimson and Ogborne [16].

Gardner and Connell [8] reported the findings in 107 opioid users attending a drug dependence clinic in London between March 1968 and February 1969 in relation to clinical groups, management policy, dosage of drugs prescribed, diagnosis of dependence, and the use of biochemical tests for the presence of drugs in urine. Diagnosis and deciding maintenance doses were especially difficult. Heroin or Methadone linctus was prescribed for some patients despite a negative urine, and some of these became addicted during their attendance at the clinic. The authors considered that heroin maintenance therapy should be re-evaluated, and that this approach should be used with great caution, if at all, in young persons. Assessment of urine for the presence of drugs was a vital part of diagnosis, treatment, and a rigorous management regime. Gardner [7], reporting on deatl.s in United Kingdom opioid users between 1965 and 1969, showed that accidental overdosage and self-administered overdosage of methadone had significantly increased.

Glatt [9] reviewed the methods of prescribing methadone in England and pointed out their marked difference from the methods used in the U.S.A. In England, less oral methadone was prescribed, and four-fifths of all methadone prescribed was in injectable form.

In three papers Bewley [1, 2, 3] presented some evidence that the clinics had had a limited success in achieving some of their goals: 20% of patients who had attended were believed to have become abstinent; 40% were functioning better in terms of stability, marriage, and work; 40% were no better but remained in regular medical contact with the health service. Medical, psychological, and social measures to alleviate distress, to ameliorate some of the ill effects of addiction and deal with its complications could be easily provided because of the open access to medical facilities without any payment at the point of entry to the system.

The clinics also appeared to have been of some value as a preventive measure, since the rate of appearance of new cases had decreased markedly in the last 3 years: Perhaps the best evidence was that the number of deaths among opiate addicts, which had been increasing by 50% annually, had ceased to escalate so rapidly. One reason for the partial success of clinics may be that the image of the "junkie" has been significantly affected when opiate addicts are defined as sick rather than sinful. Regular attendance at a hospital outpatient clinic to obtain drugs is less glamorous than obtaining them illegally in a street market from another addict. Another subtle effect of having clinics is that the subject of drug addiction becomes less newsworthy, and we have seen a decrease in the amount of newsprint on the subject, with an improvement in its quality. Stern "more must be done about the pushers" articles have been succeeded by "boring" series of articles about treatment. To some extent the clinics and the attitudes toward addiction are beginning to bring back boredom to the subject—something that is highly desirable, as it enables Government to plan rationally for the future without undue pressures.

The Present

The population attending the special clinics. A virtue of the system just described is that it aids data collection and improves intelligence. Bransby [5] has studied all patients "notified"[2] by hospitals, representing two-thirds of all

---

[2] A "notified" addict would be someone who might be referred to as a "registered" addict although there is no formal registration procedure in Britain.

TABLE 1
Age When an Opiate or Methadone or Cocaine Was First Used (Where Known)

Place of birth	Number of patients	Percent of all patients	Age (years)									
			under 14	14	15	16	17	18	19	20-24	25-29	30 and over
			%	%	%	%	%	%	%	%	%	%
Males												
All patients	1562	87	0.8	1.4	7.6	14.2	16.7	16.6	12.5	23.6	5.0	1.6
England—All patients	1284	88	0.7	1.6	8.5	14.2	17.6	17.1	12.9	22.0	4.0	1.4
Began taking drugs before 1967	778		1.2	2.1	9.9	14.8	18.4	16.8	11.8	19.6	3.6	1.8
in 1967 or later	506		–	0.8	6.3	13.3	16.4	17.6	14.6	25.7	4.5	0.8
Wales, Scotland, Northern Ireland, Irish Republic	159	85	1.3	0.6	3.8	12.6	12.6	13.2	11.9	33.3	8.8	1.9
USA, Canada	56	86	1.8	–	5.4	21.4	14.3	14.3	7.1	23.2	10.7	1.8
Elsewhere and not known	63	94	–	–	1.6	12.7	11.1	15.9	11.1	31.7	11.1	4.8
Females*												
All patients	329	82	0.6	3.7	3.0	10.3	19.2	18.5	12.8	23.1	6.1	2.7
England—All patients	273	83	0.4	4.4	2.5	10.6	18.3	18.7	13.2	23.8	5.5	2.6
Began taking drugs before 1967	173		0.6	6.4	4.0	10.4	18.5	19.7	11.5	20.8	5.8	2.3
in 1967 or later	100		–	1.0	–	11.0	18.0	17.0	16.0	29.0	5.0	3.0

*The figures for other places of birth are not given because the numbers are too small.
NOTE.—From Bransby, E. R. *Health Trends* (1971), Department of Health and Social Security.

TABLE 2
Type of Opiate or Methadone or Cocaine First Used (Where Known)

Place of birth	Number of patients	Percent of all patients	Percent who first used the drug				
			Heroin	Methadone	Cocaine	Morphine	Other opiate
Male							
All patients	1,714	96	89.8	3.7	0.4	3.6	2.5
England—All patients	1,418	97	90.5	4.0	0.4	2.9	2.2
Began taking drugs							
before 1967	775		91.2	1.3	0.5	3.4	3.6
in 1967 or later	505		90.9	6.1	0.4	2.4	0.2
Wales, Scotland, Northern Ireland, Irish Republic	168	90	89.3	3.6	—	5.9	1.2
USA, Canada	62	95	80.6	—	—	12.9	6.5
Elsewhere and not known	66	99	86.4	1.5	—	4.5	7.6
Females*							
All patients	388	97	92.5	2.6	1.0	2.6	1.3
England—All patients	316	97	92.4	2.8	1.0	2.2	1.6
Began taking drugs							
before 1967	170		93.5	0.6	1.8	1.8	2.3
in 1967 or later	99		92.9	5.1	—	2.0	—

*The figures for other places of birth are not given because the numbers are too small.

NOTE.—From Bransby, E. R. *Health Trends* (1971), Department of Health and Social Security.

TABLE 5

Current* and Past Use of Drugs (2,187 Patients)

Type of drug	MALES (place of birth) England Current	In past	Never	Not known	Wales, Scotland and Northern Ireland, Irish Republic Current	In past	Never	Not known	USA and Canada Current	In past	Never	Not known	Elsewhere and not known Current	In past	Never	Not known	FEMALES (place of birth) England Current	In past	Never	Not known	Elsewhere and not known Current	In past	Never	Not known
	%	%	%	%	%	%	%	%	%	%	%	%	%	%	%	%	%	%	%	%	%	%	%	%
Heroin	90	6	2	2	92	5	1	2	94	5	–	1	89	9	–	2	91	5	3	1	89	5	3	3
Methadone	54	8	27	11	60	7	21	12	44	15	27	14	54	8	17	21	56	9	21	14	59	7	23	11
Other opiate	7	17	52	24	8	25	38	29	5	38	30	27	6	29	35	30	4	15	50	31	5	15	58	22
Cocaine	24	23	37	16	29	22	33	16	30	27	19	24	27	22	30	21	17	20	42	21	23	17	38	22
Barbiturate	21	13	47	19	23	17	40	20	21	17	35	27	27	14	37	22	28	13	33	26	20	22	40	18
Nonbarbiturate sedative/hypnotic	18	12	47	23	15	15	42	28	11	14	46	29	16	11	43	30	18	12	40	30	19	8	50	23
Amphetamine	45	34	11	10	57	31	6	6	30	19	29	22	46	25	18	11	52	32	8	8	39	27	20	14
Amphetamine/ barbiturate																								
proprietary tablet	14	49	21	16	17	44	20	19	3	25	45	27	13	28	35	24	15	37	24	24	15	24	37	24
Hallucinogen	5	27	46	22	7	26	41	26	5	21	44	30	5	27	43	25	2	30	41	27	7	12	54	27
Cannabis	31	40	16	13	23	40	20	17	18	38	19	25	35	29	9	27	27	37	19	17	22	34	24	20

*Within one month of first attendance at hospital.

NOTE.—From Bransby, E. R. *Health Trends* (1971), Department of Health and Social Security.

147

addicts notified by all sources, during the 2-year period up to February 1970. His findings (when an opiate was first used, the type used, and the current and past use of drugs) are shown in Tables 1-3.

Another study of patients attending three drug-dependence treatment units was made by Mahon [13], who reviewed the records of 491 patients attending three clinics. He found:

1. The vast majority (85%) of the patients were under 30 years of age at the time they were first seen at a hospital as addicts.

2. The number of male addicts was 5 times that of female addicts.

3. The overwhelming majority (98%) of the patients were white, and claimed to be citizens of the United Kingdom (92%).

4. The majority (55%) came from the lower three social classes, while very few (14%) were from the upper two social classes. The remaining patients either could not be classified by him or were not in the labor force.

5. There was a substantial amount of trafficking in illicit drugs among the addict population.

6. The majority (79%) of patients in a smaller (one-third) sample were unemployed when they first attended or entered a hospital.

7. The majority (71%) of the patients in Mahon's smaller sample admitted having been arrested at least once, and the majority of these (67%) had been arrested before their first use of heroin.

8. The patients had not maintained a normal or satisfactory marital and family life.

9. The sex lives of the patients had been deleteriously affected by narcotic drugs.

10. The number (7) and percentage (1.5%) of addicted individuals in the medical profession was minimal.

11. A distinct addict subculture existed in Great Britain.

A third study of British opiate users attending treatment clinics was carried out by Blumberg [4] and his colleagues at the Addiction Research Unit, London. They studied people approaching the drug treatment centers in Greater London during 1971, and aimed to carry out a prospective study by reinterviewing them annually for 5 years. There were 210 patients in the study, 90% were born in the United Kingdom. The median present age was 21.7 years; 26% were under 20, and 72% in their 20s. Education: 59% had not completed any examinations, 22% had at least one "O"[3] level or certificate of secondary education, 4% a vocational examination, 10% at least one "A" level, 3% had entered a degree or diploma program, and the remaining 2% had a first degree or teacher's diploma. This sample does not differ markedly from the national averages for Great Britain.

---

[3] "O" levels are taken at the age of 16, A (advanced) level at the age of 18, and two or three A levels would normally be required for university entrance. A first degree would refer to a B.A. or B.Sc., a second degree to a master's or doctorate.

At the time of interview 39% were working full-time, 4% part-time, 50% were unemployed, and 7% were housewives, students, and miscellaneous. Of 205 respondents who were asked where money had come from in the 4 weeks preceding interview, 66% indicated some money had come from their own or their spouse's earnings, 49% borrowing from or sharing with friends, 38% money from relatives, 37% selling things except drugs, 34% social security, 32% selling drugs, 22% stealing. Of 100 respondents asked about the amount of contact they ever had with various social agencies, 81% indicated some contacts with the Ministry of Social Security, 70% with Probation Service, 63% with Solicitor or legal advice people, 27% Local Authority Social Worker system, 23% "Release," 18% Day Centers. Few respondents had more than three addresses in the course of the preceding 12 months. At the time of the interview 20% were married and living with their spouses, 19% lived with their steady boy or girl friend, 25% had steady boy or girl friends but were not living together, 34% had no such liaisons.

Illegal activities: 80% had had at least one conviction; 46% had had a conviction in the 12 months preceding interview; 69% had had one prior to that. Over half (52%) had been convicted of at least one drug offense, 28% in the previous year. Of 103 people asked how many convictions of any type they had had before their first "fix," 47% had had at least one.

Two groups of subjects were compared: those who were given a regular prescription for opiates (113 people) and those who were not (61 people who, for the most part, did not produce an opiate-positive urine at the time). (In 36 cases a decision was still pending.) People who were given such a prescription were likely to have been using more illicit heroin or methadone than were people who were not given an opiate prescription, and the prescription given was usually a small quantity of methadone. Significantly higher rates of unemployment, illegal activities, and physical complications were demonstrated in the group that did *not* receive a regular opiate prescription.

Table 4 shows some differences between the groups that did and did not receive a prescription for opiates; Table 5 shows the frequencies of physcial complications.

There is some evidence that the clinic system is of value and helped to contain the problem:

1. The rate at which new cases have appeared has been much lower than before the clinics were set up.
2. The overall death rate of opiate addicts has ceased to increase as rapidly as it did in the 1960s.
3. The clinics are a source of information and expertise in the treatment of opiate dependence.
4. The clinics also make it possible for treatments to be rationally assessed—when necessary by randomized controlled trials.
5. No other system so easily provides acceptable, free, open access to medical and social facilities for patients who are unmotivated or have been thrown out of other programs.

6. Some patients have been helped to abstain entirely from drug use. Others have been able to lead more stable lives despite continuing use of opiates.

TABLE 4

Characteristics of Drug Use: Differences between the
Prescription and No-Prescription Groups

Characteristics and drug	Prescription	No-Prescription
Frequency, amphetamines[a]	1.2	1.8
Frequency, methadone ampoules	3.8	2.8
Frequency, sleepers and tranquilizers[b]	1.4	1.8
Frequency, psychedelics	1.1	1.6
Liking, heroin[c]	4.7	4.1
Need, amphetamines[a]	1.2	1.6
Need, methadone ampoules	2.9	2.3
Need, opiates other than heroin and methadone	2.0	1.4
Need, sleepers and tranquilizers	1.4	1.8
Obtainability, heroin[c]	4.1	3.6
Obtainability, methedrine ampoules	1.3	1.8

NOTE.—Frequency is measured on a scale ranging from 1 (not taken in the past 4 weeks) to 5 (taken daily). The liking scale ranges from 1 (dislike) to 5 (like a lot). The need scale ranges from 1 (no need) to 4 (strong need). The obtainability scale ranges from 1 (very difficult to obtain) to 5 (very easy). All entries are mean values for those respondents who have at least tried the drug in question.

[a]The means refer to oral amphetamines. Figures for injected amphetamines are similar, except that frequency is even greater for the No-Prescription Group (who also have significantly greater liking than the Prescription Group).

[b]Means refers to injected sleepers and tranquilizers, oral being used more frequently and disliked less by both groups.

[c]Means refer to English heroin, but the figures for Chinese heroin are similar except as follows. Chinese heroin was used more frequently—and was needed more—by the Prescription Group than by the No-Prescription Group; and both groups found it easier to obtain than English heroin.

NOTE.—From Blumberg, H. H. et al. (1972), Addiction Research Unit, London.

TABLE 5
Frequencies of Physical Complications

Complication	Past year		Prior	
	No-Prescription	Prescription	No-Prescription	Prescription
Septicaemia	10 (17%)	6 (5%)	8 (13%)	8 (8%)
Hepatitis	6 (10%)	21 (19%)	9 (15%)	29 (26%)
Abcesses	23 (39%)	22[a](20%)	12 (20%)	30 (29%)
Overdose	25 (43%)	38 (34%)	28 (47%)	40 (36%)
Other injury or disease	17 (30%)	15[b](14%)	31 (54%)	35[c] (32%)
Drug-related hospitalizations	25 (42%)	28[d](25%)	21 (35%)	27 (24%)
Nondrug hospitalizations[e]	5 (9%)	8 (8%)	16 (27%)	53[f](48%)

NOTE.—Frequencies refer to the number of respondents who have had a particular complication at least once in the relevant time period. Percentages are based on the total number in the No-Prescription–or Prescription–group for whom there was a clear positive or negative response. The following significance tests are based on differences in incidence between the Prescription and No-Prescription groups.

[a] $2 = 6.12, p < .02.$
[b] $2 = 5.87, p > .02.$
[c] $2 = 7.77, p > .01.$
[d] $2 = 4.35, p > .02.$
[e] Excluding respondents who had any drug-related hospitalizations in the particular time period.
[f] $2 = 6.32, p > .02.$

NOTE.—From Blumberg, H. H. et al. (1972), Addiction Research Unit, London.

TABLE 6

United Kingdom Statistics of Drug Addiction and Criminal Offenses Involving Drugs

Year	1958	1959	1960	1961	1962	1963	1964	1965	1966	1967	1968	1969* Year total	1969* As at Dec. 31, 1969
Total number of drug addicts	442	454	437	470	532	635	753	927	1,349	1,729	2,782	2,881	1,466
Drugs†													
No. taking heroin	62	68	94	132	175	237	342	521	899	1,299	2,240	1,417	499
No. taking methadone	12	60	68	59	54	55	61	72	156	243	486	1,687	1,011
No. taking cocaine	25	30	52	84	112	171	211	311	443	462	564	311	81
No. taking morphine	205	204	177	168	157	172	162	160	178	158	198	345	111
No. taking pethidine	117	116	98	105	112	107	128	102	131	112	120	128	83
Origin													
No. of therapeutic origin	349	344	309	263	312	355	368	344	351	313	306	289	247
No. of nontherapeutic origin	68	98	122	159	212	270	372	580	982	1,385	2,420	2,533	1,196
No. of unknown origin	25	12	6	18	8	10	13	3	16	31	56	59	23
Ages													
Under 20 years	—	—	1	2	3	17	40	145	329	395	764	637	224
Taking heroin‡	—	—	1	2	3	17	40	134	317	381	709	598	221

20–34 years	—	50	62	94	132	184	257	347	558	906	1,530	1,789	897
Taking heroin‡	—	35	52	87	126	162	219	319	479	827	1,390	1,709	872
35–49 years	—	92	91	95	107	128	138	134	162	142	146	174	116
Taking heroin‡	—	7	14	19	24	38	61	52	83	66	78	101	69
50 years and older	—	278	267	272	274	298	311	291	286	279	260	241	204
Taking heroin‡	—	26	27	24	22	20	22	16	20	24	20	46	40
Age unknown	—	34	16	7	16	8	7	10	14	7	82	40	25
Taking heroin‡	—	—	—	—	—	—	—	—	—	1	43	26	13
Sex													
No. of male addicts	197	196	195	223	262	339	409	558	886	1,262	2,161	2,295	1,067
No. of female addicts	245	258	242	247	270	296	344	369	463	467	621	586	399
Professional classes (medical or allied)													
Total number	74	68	63	61	57	56	58	45	54	56	43	43	26

*It will be seen that the statistical data for 1969 is presented differently from that of the preceding years. Previously these statistics have been based on the total number of addicts coming to the notice of the Home Office during the course of the year. New recording procedures have made it possible to give details of those addicts known to have been receiving supplies of drugs at the end of the year, as well as the total number of cases coming to notice during the year.

†These figures refer to drugs used alone or in combination with other drugs. Thus an addict using both heroin and cocaine will be included under both drugs, and it must be pointed out that all but a handful of the cocaine addicts shown are also using heroin.

‡For 1969 this figure is for addicts to *heroin and/or methadone*. The reason for this is that, as a result of a deliberate policy adopted by hospital clinics in the treatment of heroin addiction of weaning patients from heroin onto methadone; methadone has supplanted heroin as the drug most commonly used by addicts.

Produced by: Drugs Branch, Home Office, Romney House, Marsham Street, London SW1.

TABLE 7
United Kingdom Drug Abuse Statistics

Drug addicts	1970		1971	
	Year total	As at 12/31/70	Year total	As at 12/31/71
Total number	2,661	1,430	2,769	1,555
Drugs†				
No. taking heroin	914	437	959	385
No. taking methadone	1,820	992	1,927	1,160
No. taking cocaine	198	57	178	58
No. taking morphine	346	105	346	103
No. taking pethidine	122	80	135	73
Origin				
No. of therapeutic origin	295	231	265	218
No. of nontherapeutic origin	2,321	1,177	2,457	1,313
No. of unknown origin	45	22	47	24
Ages				
Under 20	405	142	338	118
Taking heroin*	365	136	304	111
20-34	1,813	959	2,010	1,123
Taking heroin*	1,705	921	1,912	1,088
35-49	158	112	156	112
Taking heroin*	95	69	94	73
50 and over	253	195	226	179
Taking heroin*	50	39	47	35
Age unknown	32	22	39	23
Taking heroin*	18	10	19	9
Sex				
No. of male addicts	2,071	1,053	2,134	1,135
No. of female addicts	590	377	635	420
Professional classes (medical or allied) Total number	38	26	44	22

NOTE.–Home Office. (1972) London.

TABLE 8

Ages of "Under 20" Addicts Known
to Home Office

Year	14	15	16	17	18	19	Total
1960	–	–	–	–	–	1	1
1961	–	–	–	–	1	1	2
1962	–	–	1	–	–	2	3
1963	–	–	2	2	2	11	17
1964	1	–	1	8	11	19	40
1965	–	8	5	19	42	71	145
1966	1	17	26	68	111	106	329
1967	–	3	38	82	100	172	395
1968	–	10	40	141	274	299	764
1969 Total	–	–	24	83	218	312	637
12/31/69	–	–	6	33	73	112	224
1970 Total	–	1	9	49	117	229	405
12/31/70	–	1	1	18	30	92	142
1971 Total	–	–	10	45	114	169	338
12/31/71	–	–	2	13	34	69	118

NOTE.–Home Office. (1972) London.

7. Clinics provide treatment for medical, psychological, and social complications, and are a useful access point to medical and social care.

The situation at the end of 1971. The number of narcotic drug addicts in the United Kingdom known by the Home Office to be receiving narcotic drugs as of December 31, 1971, was 1,555 [10].

This figure was based upon statutory notifications under the Dangerous Drugs (Notification of Addicts) Regulations 1968, which required doctors to notify particulars of addicts whom they attended, and upon the examination of prescription records.

The number of addicts represented an increase of 125 (or 8.7%) over the total of 1,430 for 1970.

The 1971 figure comprised:

1,161 addicts receiving methadone (of whom 229 were also receiving heroin);
156 addicts receiving heroin (either alone or in combination with drugs other than methadone);
238 addicts receiving drugs other than methadone or heroin (for the main part, morphine or pethidine) whose addiction was mostly of therapeutic origin.

For comparison, the 1970 figure comprised:
992 addicts receiving methadone (of whom 254 were also receiving heroin);
183 addicts receiving heroin (either alone or in combination with drugs other than methadone);

TABLE 9
Classification of Narcotic Drug Addicts as of
12/31/71 by Age, Sex, and Drug

Age	Methadone			Heroin			Other Drugs		
	Male	Female	Total	Male	Female	Total	Male	Female	Total
Under 15	–	–	–	–	–	–	–	–	–
15	–	–	–	–	–	–	–	–	–
16	1	1	2	–	–	–	–	–	–
17	6	4	10	3	–	3	–	–	–
18	21	8	29	3	–	3	–	2	2
19	48	13	61	3	–	3	4	1	5
20	73	19	92	5	2	7	1	2	3
21	122	24	146	8	–	8	2	–	2
22	119	20	139	9	4	13	4	–	4
23	128	26	154	6	2	8	2	1	3
24	100	23	123	14	2	16	3	1	4
25	61	17	78	9	2	11	2	–	2
26	44	15	59	5	2	7	2	1	3
27	39	11	50	7	1	8	–	1	1
28	19	12	31	7	2	9	1	1	2
29	17	7	24	1	2	3	1	–	1
30	20	6	26	4	1	5	1	–	1
31	15	1	16	4	3	7	1	–	1
32	14	3	17	5	–	5	2	2	4
33	7	5	12	1	1	2	–	1	1
34	7	1	8	5	–	5	2	–	2
35 to 49	34	15	49	15	9	24	21	18	39
50 & over	14	12	26	5	4	9	46	98	144
Unknown	5	4	9	–	–	–	7	7	14
Totals	914	247	1,161[+]	119	37	156[†]	102	136	238

[+]Includes 229 addicts receiving heroin as well as methadone.
[†]Excludes 229 addicts receiving methadone as well as heroin.
NOTE.–Home Office. (1972) London.

255 addicts receiving drugs other than methadone or heroin (for the main part, morphine or pethidine) whose addiction was mostly of therapeutic origin.

The total number of addicts known to be receiving heroin at the end of 1971 was 385, compared with 437 at the end of 1970.

Convictions in 1971 for offenses involving drugs controlled under the Dangerous Drugs Act 1965 (e.g., heroin, cocaine, opium, and cannabis) numbered 10,844 (8,800 in 1970). These resulted from 12,293 prosecutions (9,897 in 1970). Cannabis accounted for 9,219 convictions (7,520 in 1970).

TABLE 10

Offenses Involving Drugs Controlled Under
Dangerous Drugs Act, 1965

Year	Cannabis	Opium	Manufactured drugs	Drugs (prevention of misuse) Act 1964
1945	4	206	20	
1946	11	65	27	
1947	46	76	65	
1948	51	78	48	
1949	61	52	56	
1950	86	41	42	
1951	132	64	47	
1952	98	62	48	
1953	88	47	44	
1954	144	28	47	
1955	115	17	37	
1956	103	12	37	
1957	51	9	30	
1958	99	8	41	
1959	185	18	26	
1960	235	15	28	
1961	288	15	61	
1962	588	16	71	
1963	663	20	63	
1964	544	14	101	
1965	626	13	128	958*
1966	1,119	36	242	1,216
1967	2,393	58	573	2,486
1968	3,071	73	1,099	2,957
1969	4,683	53	1,359	3,762
1970	7,520	66	1,214	3,885
1971	9,219	55	1,570	5,516

NOTE.–From 1945 to 1953 inclusive the figures relate to prosecutions. From 1954 onwards the figures relate to convictions.

*This figure is in respect of the period 31 October 1964 to 31 December 1965.

NOTE.–Home Office. (1972) London.

TABLE 11

1971 Summary of Convictions Involving Drugs Controlled Under the Dangerous Drugs Act, 1965

Drug	Unlawful possession	Unlawful supply	Unlawful procuring	Unlawful import	Premises offenses	Larceny	Other offenses	Totals
Opium	40	2	–	5	2	6	–	55
Cannabis	7,837	394	90	224	474	–	200	9,219
Heroin	439	54	15	–	–	71	1	580
Cocaine	48	6	1	1	–	70	–	126
Other drugs	379	55	69	1	–	268	92	864
Totals	8,743	511	175	231	476	415	293	10,844

Summary of Convictions Involving Drugs Controlled Under the Drugs (Prevention of Misuse) Act, 1964

Drug	Unlawful possession	Larceny	Other offenses	Totals
LSD	1,576	4	21	1,601
Other drugs	2,707	808	400	3,915
Totals	4,283	812	421	5,516

NOTE.–Home Office. (1972) London.

158

TABLE 12

Ages of Persons Found Guilty of an
Offense Involving Drugs

Ages	1970	1971
Under 14	10	23
14 and under 17	451	575
17 and under 21	4,234	5,237
21 and over	4,465	5,877
All ages	9,160	11,712

Persons Found Guilty of Offenses
Involving Drugs*

Drug	1970	1971
Raw opium	25	19
Prepared opium	32	33
Heroin	226	500
Cannabis	759	1,808
Cannabis resin	5,880	6,290
Cannabis plant	43	114
Cocaine	112	107
Other drugs controlled under the Dangerous Drugs Act 1965	577	594
Lysergide (LSD 25)	744	1,537
Other drugs controlled under the Drugs (Prevention of Misuse) Act 1964	2,181	2,810

*A number of persons were found guilty of several offenses involving either the same or different types of drugs.
NOTE.—Home Office. (1972) London.

Convictions in 1971 for offenses involving drugs controlled under the Drugs (Prevention of Misuse) Act 1964, which included amphetamines and hallucinogens such as LSD, numbered 5,516, of which 1,601 were for LSD offenses. In 1970, convictions totaled 3,885 (757 for LSD offenses).

The number of persons found guilty of offenses involving drugs controlled under these Acts was 11,712; the corresponding figure for 1970 was 9,160.

Table 6 shows United Kingdom statistics of drug addiction and criminal offenses involving drugs, from 1958 to 1969. Table 7 shows the 1970 and 1971 figures, Table 8 shows the ages of "under 20" addicts known to the Home Office, and Table 9 classifies narcotic drug addicts by age, sex, and drug. Tables 10-12 show figures relating to drug offenses.

The Future

In Britain it is likely that the future will be in some way similar to the present. The following principles with respect to treatment, for example, are unlikely to change:

1. An illness is any condition treated by doctors.
2. If all methods to deal with deviant behavior are equally unsuccessful, the medical aim may be the most humane.
3. Since the feckless and irresponsible are more likely to use drugs and develop complications for this use, doctors should be aware of their responsibilities, and the responsibility for dealing with tiresome (to the doctor) patients should not be avoided. Making a doctor responsible for a particular population or area, as can be done in the National Health Service, is a way of achieving this.
4. Since much illness is chronic and untreatable, alleviation and continuing support may be more important than curative programs.
5. We must learn to live with the casualties of our society, and drug casualties are one such group.
6. There are advantages in using a medical model for addiction, as sickness is generally less attractive than sin.

REFERENCES

1. Bewley, T. H. The treatment of opiate addicts in the United Kingdom (1968-1971), (unpublished report).
2. Bewley, T. H., James, I. P., LeFevre, C., Maddocks, P., & Mahon, T. Maintenance treatment of narcotic addicts. *International Journal of the Addictions,* 7(4), 597-611, 1972.
3. Bewley, T. H., James, I. P., & Mahon, T. Evaluation of the effectiveness of prescribing clinics for narcotic addicts in the United Kingdom(1968-1970). In C. J. D. Zarafonetis (Ed.), *Report of the International Symposium on Drug Abuse (Ann Arbor, 1970).* Philadelphia: Lea and Febiger, 1972.
4. Blumberg, H. H., Cohen, S. D., Dronfield, B. E., Mordecai, E. A., Roberts, J. C., & Hawks, D. British Opiate Users. 1. People approaching London Drug Treatment Centres. 11. Differences between those given an opiate script and those not given one, *International Journal of the Addictions,* in press.
5. Bransby, E. R. A study of patients notified by hospitals as addicted to drugs. *Health Trends,* 3(4), 75-78, 1971.
6. *Dangerous Drugs Act 1967.* London: H.M.S.O., 1967.
7. Gardner, R. Death in United Kingdom opioid users 1965-1969. *Lancet,* 2, 650-653, 1970.
8. Gardner, R., & Connell, P. H. One year's experience in a drug dependence clinic. *Lancet,* 2, 455-458, 1970.
9. Glatt, M. M. Present-day methadone prescribing in England. *International Journal of the Addictions,* 7, 173-177, 1972.

10. Home Office Reports. *Reports to the United Nations on the workings of the International Treaties on Narcotic Drugs.* London: H.M.S.O., 1969–1972.
11. Interdepartmental Committee. *Drug addiction. Report of the Interdepartmental Committee.* London: H.M.S.O., 1961.
12. Interdepartmental Committee. *Drug addiction. Second Report of the Interdepartmental Committee.* London: H.M.S.O., 1965.
13. Mahon, T. A. An exploratory study of hospitalised narcotic addicts in Great Britain. *Acta Psychiatrica.* Scandinavica Supplement 227. Copenhagen: Munksgaard, 1971.
14. Ministry of Health. *Report of the Departmental Committee on Morphine and Heroin Addiction* (Rolleston report). London: H.M.S.O., 1926.
15. Spear, H. B. The growth of heroin addiction in the United Kingdom. *British Journal of Addiction,* **64,** 245–255, 1969.
16. Stimson, G. V., & Ogborne, H. C. A survey of a representative sample of addicts prescribed heroin at London clinics. *Bulletin of Narcotics,* **22**(4), 13–22, 1970.

TECHNOLOGY AND THE
TREATMENT OF ADDICTION

Matthew P. Dumont
Massachusetts Department of Mental Health

Let us assume a hypothetical situation of a society, not unlike ours, which has recognized suicidal behavior as a matter of grave concern and a cause for major governmental initiative. It has decided to concentrate its concern on wrist slashing. The reason for that decision is unclear in view of the fact that most successful suicides resort to other modes, but wrist slashing can be fatal as well as messy. Moreover, the mixture of horror and fascination it arouses in the public mind can be exploited for the purpose of launching expensive new programs at a time of austerity.

The leader of the nation declares wrist slashing to be public enemy number one, and a bold and comprehensive program is designed with unprecedented authority to cut through the usual middle-managerial passive-aggressive mechanisms of government. Agencies that could not cooperate on such issues as transportation, housing, employment, health care, malnutrition, pollution, and war are told that they *shall* cooperate on wrist slashing or "heads will roll." Prevention of wrist slashing is given a high priority, and TV spots, billboards, and magazines purport to be doing a public service in suicide prevention by showing pictures of young people slashing their wrists. The precise angle and depth of the razor blade for the most lethal cut is carefully displayed. Former wrist slashers are hired to appear on television, in classrooms, and in Rotary Club halls to show their scars, describe the exquisite pain of their cutting experience, and express their gratitude for being alive today to warn children away from the purveyors of razor blades.

While wrist slashing itself is defined as a sickness, the possession of razor blades is declared a felony. The manufacture and sale of razor blades is considered the most heinous crime imaginable and at every level of government major increases are provided in police manpower to crack down on the blade market. It soon becomes clear that wrist slashers do not volunteer for treatment before, during, or after their slashing, and indeed do not appear to want treatment. A major expansion of treatment programs must rely on a process of involuntary commitments to justify their existence. One treatment appears to be particularly attractive to the patients, however. It involves the legal dispensation of surgical scalpel blades by governmentally approved and medically controlled clinics. When these clinics are well run, the patient is subjected to a carefully prescribed regimen of nurse-administered wrist cuts of gradually increasing depth, the wrists becoming so scarified that no pain is felt and no blood drawn. At that point, the patient may have his own scalpel blades, and having been labeled as a wrist slasher he is urged to lead as normal a life as possible.

In poorly run clinics, or in the hands of unscrupulous or disingenuous practitioners, blades are administered promiscuously with the result that surgical scalpel blades become a favored instrument for wrist slashing. When this becomes apparent, more rigorous government supervision of such clinics is called for at the same time that a major expansion is anticipated. New measures are suggested, including a national or regional registry of all wrist slashers as a way of controlling the diversion of scalpel blades and, incidentally, for obtaining some epidemiological data.

The top and virtually exclusive priority for basic research is chosen to be the elaboration of wrist guards for known slashers. It is suggested that mass screening techniques in schools and other institutions may show up individuals who are wrist-slashing-prone, and such persons may have wrist guards imposed upon them to prevent them from actually cutting themselves.

Even strained analogies such as this one may be helpful for the synthesis of general principles. There is some silliness in this hypothetical situation. While there may be some shared characteristics, perhaps even distinguishing ones, among wrist slashers, it is silly to assume that if someone is considering suicide he or she is not likely to choose some other mode. It is even sillier to try to control the production and distribution of razor blades, or to adopt prosecution for illegal possession as a presumed deterrent. Silliest of all is to develop a whole juggernaut of medical and industrial technology to make wrist slashing a less effective way of committing suicide.

The reflexive American response to any problem is technology. This has even been true when the problems are themselves the products of technology. We create ever more elaborate mechanisms to deal with the unforeseen consequences of a previous array of elaborate mechanisms.

Most of society's problems are ecological, in the sense that they do not exist in a well-circumscribed module of behavior. There are complex interplays of cultural, social, biological, and psychological forces whose shifting influences run over, through, and around us like lights at a rock festival. To do one thing in an ecological system is not possible, and it is difficult to anticipate second-order and third-order consequences. The technological response, however, has to assume that a social problem can be repaired like a carburetor. It must arbitrarily define boundaries because it is impatient with the mysteries of disappearing interfaces. It can only become increasingly efficient for subordinate goals, because superordinate ones defy technological capacities. Technology can, for example, get us to the moon but much less effectively tell us whether or not we should go. It can create "smart bombs" but not peace treaties. It can deal only with what is possible without assessing what is worthwhile. And technology, insecure with moral and philosophical questions, finally creates its own value system. "Because something can be done, it should be done."

The technological mentality has shown itself in pure culture in its response to drug abuse. It has defined its arena in terms of heroin addiction—when stamping out the intravenous use of heroin might be like stepping in a globule of mercury. Despite the more extensive (and more dangerous) resort to alcohol and barbiturates by drug abusers, we have seen an almost single-minded preoccupation with the physical aspects of heroin use in the current national drug control program. What has been gained if a population of heroin users is saturated with methadone, cyclazocine, or naloxone, deconditioned to needle use by aversive techniques, rendered forgetful by cingulotomies or E.C.T. or CO_2 therapy, threatened with draconian penalties for recidivism, and now merely switches to chronic alcoholism or barbiturate addiction?

We know that the "sick role," whether achieved or ascribed, carries with it a set of behaviors, perceptions, and expectations vastly different from those within and about the same individuals before their assumption of that role. The most marked characteristic of this role is a sense of helplessness and dependency, a denial of free choice now adopted by "the patient." What is frequently seen as lack of "motivation" for treatment in the addict is in fact his reluctance to adopt the sick role. In this connection, a major difference between medical models of approaching addiction and the various self-help approaches is that the latter assume that the use or nonuse of drugs, even after physiological addiction, is always a deliberate and conscious decision. The premise of the therapeutic community is that in the face of a broader array of options the addict will choose a behavior pattern of honesty, responsibility, and mutuality after he has experienced them and learned them to be less chimerical than he previously thought. It remains a matter of choice; it is not the technique—as in a medical intervention—but the individual which succeeds or fails.

The White House program of research in drug abuse is focusing almost exclusively on the neurochemical and pharmacological dimension of heroin addiction. We should certainly welcome some new biochemical insights into addictive behavior, but with such a heavy preoccupation with the biochemical and pharmacological we are led to wonder if some very large eggs are being forced into one very small basket.

It is entirely possible that there is something neurochemically unique about the heroin addict. Ultimately all behavior is neurochemically mediated, and the difference between depressive and manic behavior, between schizophrenic and neurotic behavior, and, for all we know, between Democratic and Republican behavior is neurochemical.

The real issues have to do with whether or not the neurochemical distinctions are unique and salient, and what the consequences are of a focus on those distinctions.

If in dealing with the schizophrenic, for example, we were to be concerned with biochemical issues only, we would ignore the expectations and institutional pressures that the "social breakdown syndrome" involves. Whatever biochemical origins there are to schizophrenia, the most disabling aspects of the illness often emerge only after the imposition of patienthood and the "closed ranks" phenomenon that follows.

We are about to engage drug abuse with that kind of shortsighted reductional state of mind. Suppose it turns out that the most important thing one can do for an addict is find him a meaningful job. Suppose the great majority of employers do not believe addicts can be rehabilitated. What would be the consequences of a massive program of early case-finding, particularly involving "mass screening in schools and other institutions"? They could be more destructive than addiction itself. But of course we will not know. This is not considered an important issue for research in the White House. And a feeble effort of a few staff members in the Special Action Office for Drug Abuse Prevention to develop a vocational rehabilitation program for addicts must go begging to other federal agencies, while close to a billion dollars is channeled to treatment programs of questionable value and research on antagonists.

What is even more outrageous is that under the direction of the White House, the Office of Economic Opportunity, having done such a splendid job in defeating poverty, is turning its capacities in the direction of the "drug menace" by putting money into methadone maintenance programs with more alacrity than it ever demonstrated in finding jobs for the poor.

There may be other unforeseen second-order consequences to this focus on the pharmacological in the national drug program. It has been suggested that one reason for the widespread use of drugs among the young is a certain kind of ambience which supports that behavior [1]. We live in a pill-taking culture, it has been said, where all disease, discomfort, and dissatisfaction can be corrected by pharmacology [2]. We also live in an environment in which no human problem shall be considered insoluble, where no truths shall be mysterious or spiritual but all shall be capable of analysis and mechanical control. It is possible that this environmental press, in conjunction with other variables, acts as an inducement to experimentation with drugs. If this is so, the emphasis on methadone and opiate antagonists in the national program may be supporting to an environmental set which it might want to counteract.

In presenting his highest priority in research to be in opiate antagonists, the Director of the White House Special Action Office announced that the major advantage of these agents may not be in treating confirmed heroin addicts but in preventing "experimenters" from becoming addicts. "American medicine," he said, "now has the knowledge to detect heroin use by means of inexpensive, reliable, and rapid tests. Some medical or community groups might elect to use such techniques in high risk populations . . . and thereby discover heroin experimenters before they become addicted. Once diagnosed, these early potential addicts could be 'temporarily immunized' by daily treatment with antagonists [6]."

I have elsewhere [3, 4, 5] discussed some of the civil-libertarian aspects of the current national drug abuse control program. But one small item needs constant reemphasis. Threats to freedom will come in more subtle and arcane forms hereafter. The *auto-da-fè* and the concentration camp are cumbersome and inelegant ways to deal with enemies of a social order. Keeping track of individual offenders is expensive and inefficient in a complex and pluralistic system. There remain some old-fashioned liberal sensibilities here and there that make overt persecution of undesirables difficult. There is no reason to believe that the scapegoating of minority groups or the elimination of political enemies will stop. What is likely to happen is a conceptual blurring between persecution and treatment, with new forms of control based on predictors of group behavior rather than individual monitoring systems.

The White House seems to have a special affinity for early predictors of troublesome behavior in "high risk groups." Delinquency-prone, protest-prone, civil-disobedience-prone, and addiction-prone behavior is an irresistible arena of research and development for a mentality "fed up with permissiveness." That these various trouble-prone groups tend to overlap on the young or the black or the unemployed makes all this doubly attractive.

Middle-managers, technicians, and scientists have a well-established capacity to deny responsibility for the social consequences of the knowledge they generate and the information they manage. But now there are too many of them working too close to sources of power in increasingly large institutions with constantly growing authority over our lives. Any discussion of registries, predictors, and early identifiers of high risk groups must be seen in the context of a relentless movement in the direction of bureaucratic control of individual behavior based on actuarial data. It is too late to be cavalier and defensive. It is too late to be smug and self-righteous. It is too late to be thoughtlessly scientistic. The Great American Center has been given an enormous mandate to intolerance. Scientists have a special responsibility to avoid being its agents.

We need to engage the problem of drug abuse with a whole new system of questions which will involve at least three painful states of mind: (*a*) humility; (*b*) fearlessness in the face of profound social change, and (*c*) respect for what I will have to call, for the moment, "spirituality." Let me be a bit more specific.

Humility.   Let's face it. We may already be a dead profession. Too many of our colleagues are thrashing around with an "anything goes" attitude towards treatment. A half century after Freud told us that abreaction in itself is not therapeutic, some of us are calling anything and everything curative merely because it can arouse an intense emotional reaction. Those who continue to labor in the private fields of one-to-one psychotherapy are finding it more difficult to find the bread-and-butter clientele of young, middle-class, insight-oriented anxiety hysterics. During a recession psychotherapy becomes a luxury, and such patients are becoming attracted to sensitivity groups, massage groups, meditation groups, or whatever. No longer in a bullish market, psychotherapists have emerged as the entrepreneurs we always were, now ready to provide whatever touchy-feely, screamy-meany, or wowsy-boom sex therapy our patients are willing to purchase. Some of our brotherhood are actually doing this in the context of profit-making corporations, so that if things really get big they won't be locked out of the finger-licking underside of the American Dream.

Institutional psychiatry, we have known for some time now, has been all but catastrophic. The boldness and vision of the community mental health movement has become a feeble and ineffectual effort to remedy our past mistakes. Our preoccupation with psychopathology, our social class, cultural, and sexual biases, and our reliance on aggressive technologies have destroyed some of our patients. The real lesson of the Eagleton affair is not that mental illness carries political liability but that *patienthood* does.

To approach the drug abuser with traditional psychiatric techniques is to learn just how effective those techniques are. Time here for a chilling pause.

Fearlessness in the face of social change. By and large we have adopted the values of cops, the sensibilities of liberals, and the technologies of physicians. The result has been a mishmash of interventions which are nothing less than behavioral trade-offs, social controls masquerading as therapies.

Only the youngest of our profession appear to understand how different the world is now than it was a short while ago. Most of us can neither understand nor appreciate what has happened to the family, to individualism, to organizational life, to sexuality, and to politics. Here, too, drug abuse may invoke a nemesis to psychiatry. Once we learn how pervasive and how compelling are mind-altering drugs we may begin to recognize that behaviors which we have been dismissing as pathological are becoming *normative*.

There is a particular lesson here for those of our colleagues least anxious to learn it; the aggressive ones who like to push shock buttons or cut neurons or develop operant conditioning programs. We really do not know where we want to go with our patients, and they do not know where they want to go themselves. We are working in an existential labyrinth and our techniques are getting more and more drastic. It's like speeding up when you are lost. It makes no sense.

Respect for "spirituality." The need to put quotation marks around that word expresses the disdain in which we have been taught to hold it. Psychiatry, like the rest of our world, clings to an empiricist and rationalistic tradition like a baby chimp to its mother's back. When we are forced to be imaginative, as with Freud, we have to conceive of a psychoanalytic "topography" whose components have a structure and depth suggestive of thalamic tracts and limbic systems, things one can touch and cut into. We are very uncomfortable with psychological phenomena that cannot quickly be related to the firing off of neurons, even though we may have forgotten precisely where they are.

We have trodden a narrow no-man's-land between organic and functional constructs of mentality, but our faces have always deferentially turned towards the organic, like an army passing its true flag. There was always a chill at our necks, murmurs of the magic and mysticism from our distant past. We have never even allowed ourselves to be homesick for the adorable mysteries which used to hang like a mist over the world of madness, dreams, hidden wishes, and dark fears. We became behavioral scientists, bullies of empiricism like the doctor in Bergman's film *The Magician*.

Suddenly we are surrounded by a whole generation of enchanted gardens. Zen, Yoga, Bahai, Meher Baba, Sufi—sect after sect, convert after convert, crowd after crowd, a tidal wave of chanting, dancing, meditating, fasting, proselytizing, wandering, begging boys and girls who used to fidget in Unitarian churches. And Christianity itself, now returned with a burning ferocity, a frantic, abandoned, tongue-talking ecstasy which makes priests shrug like rabbis before Hasids. Everywhere, everyone is looking for inner doors to open. In a world whose oceans have become coated with oil, whose forests have been shaved to make magazines, whose winds have become yellowed with sulphurous fumes, whose fields have become suburban developments and whose dunes have become steel plants, we have a whole generation who have chosen to look to the "other-worldly."

It has traditionally been the task of mind-altering drugs to simulate a passage to spritual realms. Tainted smoke would permit an Arab to see through flies, camels, and smoldering sand into a garden of paradise. A dark mushroom would carry an Indian from a primitive hut onto a god's lips. A shimmering leaf would wing a supplicant from a lethargic jungle to exhilarated heights.

The treatment of drug abuse may make us philosophers once again. It forces us to face the unknown and respect it for its grandness.

REFERENCES

1. Dumont, M. Why the young use drugs. *Social Policy,* **2**(4), November/December, 1971.
2. Dumont, M., & Lewis, D. The "magic bullet" syndrome. *Massachusetts Journal of Mental Health,* **2**(2), Winter, 1972.
3. Dumont, M. The politics of drugs: The junkie as political enemy. *Social Policy*, **3**(2), July/August, 1972.
4. Dumont, M. The computer sees the truth but waits. *American Journal* **1**(2), December, 1972.
5. Dumont, M. Civil commitment of the addict—A critical analysis. *International Yearbooks of Drug Addiction and Society,* in press.
6. *HEW News.* Rockville, Md., July 7, 1972.

SECTION 2
INTRODUCTION

Henry Brill
Pilgrim State Hospital
West Brentwood, New York

The last few years have seen important advances in the treatment of opiate dependence, but this still remains a rapidly changing field marked by much controversy. Today one even hears certain demands that drug studies be redirected to become undertakings for social and political change. Such demands are undoubtedly well-intentioned, and they are in line with many contemporary sociopolitical trends, but they threaten the integrity of drug dependence research and indeed of biological research generally. If followed, they can be expected to debase research without achieving the stated goal of constructive social change. Those who seek to politicize research in this way attack current drug research as a tool of the military-industrial medical establishment; they impugn the motivations and ethics of scientists and condemn current techniques and procedures. Such attacks seem to come from a relatively few individuals within professional ranks. Therefore, they might be seen as nothing more than an expression of a healthy self-criticism, distressing in tone but not out of place at the present time when all values are being critically re-examined and many of them are being reversed.

But there is more. Mixed with the criticism are demands that research in drug addiction and abuse should be measured primarily, if not solely, by certain sociopolitical standards. Such demands are meant literally and not metaphorically. They are not a conscious hyperbole. They must be recognized for what they are and rejected honestly and flatly. To do less is to leave the impression that they have a basic validity, whereas both experience and logic show that the opposite is true. History shows that this has been tried before. Biological research has been subordinated to sociopolitical tests in the past, and the results have been pernicious politics and pseudoscientific research. In Communist

Russia, Marxist-Leninist dialectical materialism was used as a test for scientific relevance, and this produced Lysenkoism, a catastrophe for both science and society. In Nazi Germany, political restrictions of an opposite sort did great damage to that country and its science. By all accounts Communist China suffered in the same way when it placed its medical technologists at forced labor to meet its own special social and political standards.

If we need more examples, they can be found scattered throughout the history of science. They all point to the same conclusion, namely, that politics and science cannot be mixed.

The proposals for politicizing drug research are as weak logically as they are historically. The overriding fact is that better methods of prevention and treatment are desperately needed, and these can come only through the application of the kind of expertise possessed by trained scientists. To force them by pressure tactics to redirect their energies toward political action would be to destroy their specific usefulness.

In examining the logic of this assault on drug research, one must not be distracted by the personal attacks with which they are punctuated. The temptation is to reply in kind and to examine the motives and ethics of the attackers equally with those of the attacked. Such an exchange would be amusing to onlookers, but it would not get at basic issues. The fundamental flaw in Lysenkoism was not Lysenko's personality and his political ambitions; it was the fallacy of the idea that scientific thought can be compressed into a political mold without being destroyed. To those who are persuaded to exchange their medical technology for political action and who wish to force others to do likewise, I would quote Shakespeare, "Cobbler stick to your last."

One rational approach to the controversy is to evaluate the existing evidence bearing on the treatment of addiction. Here, direct personal communication is essential if one is to remain fully abreast of current developments. The four papers presented in this section represent such personal communication. Each is prepared by a well-known authority and is based on original work and personal experience.

The first paper is by Dr. John Ball, who reports on a field study of a series of treatment programs in Pennsylvania. He presents certain suggestions for dealing with problems which were encountered. These problems developed during a period of extremely rapid creation of new facilities and expansion of existing ones.

The growth of drug dependence programs has been paralleled by the growth of controversy about them. This is particularly true about methadone maintenance. Some writers doubt whether methadone is associated with any clinical improvement; others see improvement but attribute it entirely to nonpharmacological factors. Dr. Senay reports on a study which addresses itself to these issues. In this work he seeks to measure the effect of the drug as distinct from the rest of the treatment program, and he includes observations on methadyl acetate as well as methadone itself.

The third paper deals with narcotic antagonists. It is by Dr. Max Fink, a pioneer in this area of psychopharmacology. I know of no one who has had more experience or is better qualified to tell us about the present situation concerning the narcotic antagonists, particularly cyclazocine.

Dr. Kleber summarizes the use of narcotic antagonists as a part of a multimodality treatment program. His paper, too, is clinically oriented and describes a very carefully monitored, well-documented experience at the Drug Dependence Unit of the Connecticut Mental Health Center in New Haven.

PHASE I EVALUATION OF DRUG TREATMENT PROGRAMS IN PENNSYLVANIA[1]

John C. Ball[2]
Temple University

and

Harold Graff
Eastern Pennsylvania Psychiatric Institute

As a first step in a comprehensive plan to evaluate drug treatment programs in the Commonwealth of Pennsylvania, a research team from Temple University Health Sciences Center conducted on-site visits to all 77 programs in the state. This report analyzes the detailed survey findings.

The Field Survey Procedure

The four members of the survey team consisted of two sociologists, one psychiatrist, and one social worker.[3] Each drug treatment program was visited by at least two of the team members, and many were seen by all four. The field work was undertaken during a 12-month period ending in May of 1972. The team traveled a total of 21,486 miles during the survey period.

At each site the program director or other staff members were interviewed. A standardized interview schedule containing 60 items was employed to obtain consistent data from all the programs. In addition, a complete tour of the facility was made and, as occasion dictated, particular aspects of the program reviewed— records, medical care, administration, staffing pattern, community relations.

The overall purpose of the on-site survey was to ascertain the number and type of drug treatment programs in the Commonwealth, describe the demographic

[1] This statewide evaluation project was supported by a contract from the Department of Welfare, Commonwealth of Pennsylvania.

[2] Currently at the Special Action Office for Drug Abuse Prevention, Washington, D.C. The opinions expressed in this paper do not necessarily reflect the views of the Special Action Office.

[3] John C. Ball, PhD, Freda Adler, PhD, Frederick B. Glaser, MD, and Arthur D. Moffett, MSW.

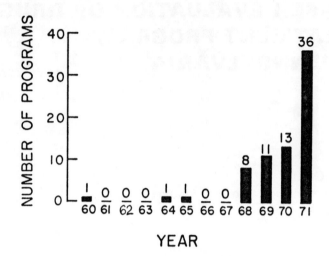

YEAR

FIG. 1. Year in which drug treatment programs were established.
Note: Not shown in Fig. 1 are the programs established during
the first months of 1972.

characteristics of drug abusers, and obtain information on the adequacy of
the treatment provided. In sum, the purpose of the project was to provide a
comprehensive delineation of "the state of the art" in Pennsylvania in 1972.
First, however, it is pertinent to briefly trace the historical development of drug
abuse programs in the state [4].

History of Drug Abuse Treatment

Most of the treatment programs for drug abusers in Pennsylvania are of recent
origin [2]. Indeed, of the 77 programs extant at the time of our field evaluation,
all but 3 were established during the past 5 years.

Figure 1 shows the number of drug treatment programs established each year.
The first program, begun in 1960 by the Pennsylvania Department of Probation
and Parole, provided counseling and social service assistance for Philadelphia
offenders who were drug abusers or addicts. Thus, the earliest emphasis was
upon compulsory rehabilitative services for hard-core opiate addicts.

The next two drug treatment programs, established by Teen Challenge in the
mid-1960s, were residential therapeutic communities with a religious orientation. The Philadelphia Teen Challenge program began in 1964 and, a year later, a
large residential farm facility was opened in Central Pennsylvania at Rehrersburg.

A major expansion of drug treatment programs occurred in 1968, when eight
new programs were established; four of these were methadone maintenance
facilities, two were residential therapeutic communities, one provided individual
counseling for drug abusers, and one stressed group therapy. As the number of

TABLE 1
Distribution of Drug-Abuse Programs, Staff and Patients by Treatment
Modality—Pennsylvania, 1972

Treatment modality	Number of programs	Number of staff	Number of patients	Percentage of patients
A. Methadone maintenance	17	213	2,816	50.5
B. Residential therapeutic community	13	147	624	11.2
C. Religious therapeutic community	7	125	175	3.1
D. Nonresidential therapeutic community	8	116	265	4.8
E. Detoxification	2	42	33	0.6
F. Individual counseling	19	82	908	16.3
G. Other modalities	11	54	757	13.6
TOTAL	77	779	5,578	100.0

treatment programs began to increase markedly, evidently quite diverse approaches to the treatment of drug abuse were being taken. During the next 3 years, in fact, 60 new programs were established in Pennsylvania to provide a diversity of treatment and rehabilitative services for drug abusers.

Major Modalities of Treatment in 1972

As both the number of drug treatment programs and the number of drug abusers receiving treatment in the Commonwealth continue to increase, it seems that most, if not all, of the major modalities of treatment are amply represented (as of late 1972) in the existing programs [3] (Table 1).

Methadone programs in Pennsylvania. At the time of our field study there were 17 methadone maintenance programs. The first four of these programs were established in 1968—two in Philadelphia, one in Pittsburgh, and one in Harrisburg. During the past 5 years, not only the number of programs but also the number of patients in these programs have increased considerably. Thus, with 50% of the patients in treatment (2,816 of 5,578), methadone maintenance is the leading modality of treatment for drug abusers in Pennsylvania.

Although the number of patients enrolled in the 17 methadone programs varies considerably, each of these clinics tends to treat more patients than do other modalities. Thus, 8 of the 17 facilities had a patient census of 100 or more, and 2 had over 500 outpatients. Indeed, these two programs—Black Action in Pittsburgh with 622 patients and the West Philadelphia Consortium with 877 patients—are the largest in the State.

The 17 methadone maintenance programs are medical in orientation and supervision. In eight programs, the director is a physician. In all programs, the treatment staff includes physicians, although usually on a part-time basis. In addition, most of the methadone clinics are located in hospitals or have special arrangements with hospitals to provide such services as physical examinations, laboratory tests, or "detoxification." A further, and perhaps paramount, reason for the medical orientation is that dispensing medication is the most frequent treatment activity and is customarily done under medical supervision. Indeed, it would not be an exaggeration to say that the dispensation of methadone is the unifying process which permeates the entire program and which gives it a medical orientation.

Residential therapeutic communities. The 13 residential therapeutic communities primarily treat the same population of heroin addicts as the methadone clinics. In the former modality, however, the treatment process is an intensive and continuing experience, as residents are under constant and active supervision. Both behavior modification techniques and psychodynamic approaches are employed. Not only are most of the staff members ex-addicts, but the absence of a professional staff is often a matter of pride. These programs are characterized by a pervasive ideological commitment on the part of staff and patients.

Religious therapeutic communities. Four of the seven religiously oriented residential treatment communities in Pennsylvania are affiliated with the national Teen Challenge Organization. The largest of these four is located on an operating farm in Berks County; the other three Teen Challenge Programs are in Philadelphia, Pittsburgh, and Harrisburg. What these rehabilitation programs emphasize is the development of work skills and the acquisition of such basic educational skills as reading, writing, and ciphering [3].

Nonresidential therapeutic communities. The ideological and behavioral orientation of these eight drug treatment programs is similar to that of the residential therapeutic communities. Both types are stringently anti-drug. Both are primarily staffed by ex-addicts. Both foster close in-group and moralistic attitudes. The nonresidential programs, however, demand less total compliance on the part of members and are more involved in community affairs and problems. They also attract a larger proportion of middle-class clients and fewer heroin addicts than their residential counterparts.

Detoxification. We found a general lack of detoxification facilities for opiate abusers throughout the state. There were only two such detoxification programs, with a total of 33 heroin addicts in treatment. Both were in Philadelphia area hospitals.

Individual counseling programs. There were 19 programs for drug abusers in which individual counseling was the principal modality of treatment; in these therapy is done primarily by professionals (social workers, graduate students, psychologists, and occasionally psychiatrists) on a one-to-one basis. In addition, some of the programs have supervised group sessions. The individual counseling centers generally resemble outpatient clinics, although the treatment atmosphere is more informal and peer-oriented. Most of the youthful clients are users of marijuana, amphetamines, barbiturates, or LSD, rather than heroin.

Other modalities of treatment. The remaining 11 programs included 6 in which outpatient group therapy was the focal point of treatment; there were 3 drop-in centers, one social action program, and one multimodality facility. In the group therapy programs, both professional and ex-addict staff serve as leaders in the treatment process. The drop-in centers, or rap houses, cater mainly to young, middle-class, "soft" drug users. The social action program used participation in neighborhood projects as the primary means of rehabilitation. The multimodality facility was primarily a methadone maintenance clinic, although efforts were afoot to expand the range of treatment alternatives.

Characteristics of Drug Abusers Receiving Treatment in Pennsylvania

There were 5,578 drug abusers in treatment within the Commonwealth at the time of our on-site evaluation of the 77 programs. In this section, the geographical distribution of these patients will be analyzed and their social characteristics delineated, in order to answer two questions: Where are the drug abusers in Pennsylvania? Who are they?

Location within the Commonwealth. Drug abusers were receiving treatment in 24 of the 67 counties of Pennsylvania in 1972 (Figure 2). Seventeen of these 24 counties were metropolitan areas (classified as Standard Metropolitan Statistical Areas by the Census Bureau), and there was a marked concentration of patients in the two principal cities—Philadelphia and Pittsburgh.

Of the 5,578 drug abusers in treatment, 46% were in Philadelphia County, and 24% in Allegheny County; the remaining 30% were located in the other 22 counties shown in Figure 2. The impact of the two large metropolitan centers upon the prevalence of drug abuse is even greater than these figures indicate, as most of the drug abusers who are not in these two cities reside in adjacent or contiguous counties. Still, the fact that most of the counties below 100,000 population have no drug abusers in treatment, while most of those with 100,000 or above have drug abusers in treatment, suggests that population density as well as proximity to the two major cities are associated with the prevalence of drug abuse.

With regard to metropolitan concentration of drug abusers, two further points are relevant. First, since most of the drug abusers in treatment (96%) are local residents, there is little support for a "drift hypothesis" to explain the

THE TREATMENT OF DRUG ABUSE IN PENNSYLVANIA

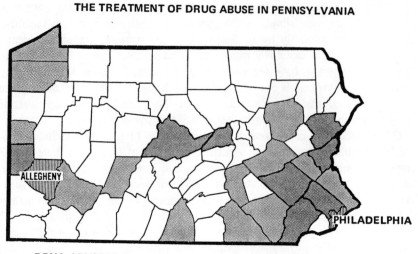

DRUG ABUSERS IN TREATMENT PER 10,000 OF POPULATION:

- 8.0 AND ABOVE . . . . HIGH RATE
- 7.9 TO 3.1 . . . . AVERAGE RATE
- 3.0 AND BELOW . . . . LOW RATE
- 0 . . . . NONE IN TREATMENT

FIG. 2. Number of drug abusers in treatment by county.

concentration of drug abusers in large metropolitan areas [1]. Second, it is necessary to analyze *rates* of drug abusers in treatment if accurate scientific statements are to be made about statewide distribution.

Rates of drug abusers in treatment. Rates of drug abusers in treatment were determined for all 67 counties by calculating the number of persons in treatment per 10,000 population. The highest rates were obtained for Philadelphia and Allegheny Counties were 13.2 and 8.2, respectively. The rate of drug abusers in treatment in Philadelphia is markedly higher than in any other part of the state.

A comparison of black and white drug abusers. The rate of drug abusers in treatment in Pennsylvania is 10 times higher for blacks than for whites. Of the 5,578 drug abusers, 45% were black and 55% were white. These rates may be compared with the 1970 racial composition of the state: of the total population (11,804,324), 91% was white and 9% was black. As might be expected, the black patients were concentrated in Philadelphia and Allegheny Counties. As was not expected, however, the black rates (the number in treatment per 10,000 population) were high in 17 counties and the highest rates were not found in the two largest cities. A plausible interpretation of this unexpected finding is that drug abuse is a major problem in most black communities throughout the Commonwealth and, secondly, that the available treatment in both Philadelphia and Pittsburgh is inadequate. The long waiting lists in these two cities support the latter interpretation.

TABLE 2

Employment Status of Drug Abusers

Status	Drug abusers	
	Number	Percent
Unemployed	3,296	59.1
Employed	1,595	28.6
Attending school	513	9.2
Attending college	174	3.1
TOTAL	5,578	100.0

Social characteristics of the drug abusers. We noted that the 5,578 drug abusers in treatment were located in 24 counties, concentrated in the two largest cities of the Commonwealth, and that the black population was overrepresented. In addition, drug abuse is primarily an indigenous problem in the sense that the vast majority of those receiving treatment are local residents. Of those in treatment, 96% were Pennsylvania residents and most of these were from the same county in which they sought treatment.

The drug abusers in treatment were a youthful population. Some 4% were 17 years of age or younger, 34% were between the ages of 18 and 20, and 59% were 21 to 30 years old; only 3% were 30 or older. The age range of all patients in treatment was from 9 to 78 years. With respect to race, the black drug abusers were older than the white—most of those over 25 were black, while most of those under 21 were white.

Most of the drug abusers in treatment were not gainfully employed, although the vast majority were in outpatient facilities. Some 59% did not have steady employment; 12% were attending public school or college; only 29% were employed (Table 2). These findings support the interpretation that persistent abuse of drugs is usually incompatible with steady employment or long-term academic achievement. At the same time, it should be recognized that drug abusers commonly seek treatment only when compelled to do so by dint of circumstances—ill health, family disruption, fear of arrest, or lack of funds. As a consequence, those in treatment may appear to be more socially impaired than they were previously.

Another indication of the social inadequacy of many youthful drug abusers is their economic dependence upon the state. Almost half (44%) of the 5,578 drug abusers in treatment in Pennsylvania were recipients of public welfare. There is, then, an association between their current drug dependence and their economic dependence.

Type of drug abused. At each of 77 treatment programs visited, we ascertained the principal drug abused by patients before admission. In 54 of the

TABLE 3

Location of 77 Treatment Facilities by Principal Drug of Abuse

Location of program	Treatment Facilities		
	Heroin	Other drugs	Total
Philadelphia County	14	–	14
Allegheny County	17	6	23
Other Counties	23	17	40
TOTAL	54	23	77

programs, heroin was the main drug of abuse. Of the other 23 programs, 12 reported that their patients were primarily polydrug abusers; 5 mentioned amphetamines; 3, marijuana; and 1, barbiturates.

In addition to the principal drug of abuse, we asked at each program which other drugs were abused. The following drugs were mentioned: heroin, morphine, methadone, amphetamines, LSD, tranquilizers, barbiturates, marijuana, hashish, mescaline, cocaine, glue, solvent, and alcohol.

A comparison of the programs in which heroin is the principal drug of abuse with the others reveals rather striking geographic and racial differences. Of the 23 polydrug abuse programs (using this term for all the nonheroin programs), 17 were outside of Philadelphia and Allegheny Counties. Conversely, 31 of the 54 programs in which heroin was the principal drug of abuse were located in these two metropolitan areas. Clearly, the heroin abusers were heavily concentrated in the two largest cities of the state, while most of the polydrug abusers were in the contiguous or outlying counties [1] (Table 3).

It is also significant that all the 23 polydrug treatment programs had a majority of white patients. There was not a single polydrug abuse program with predominantly black patients. In all the black programs, heroin was the principal drug of abuse before admission [1].

Patient and Staff Census of May 1972

Because most of the drug treatment programs were undergoing change or expansion at the time of our initial on-site visit, we decided to update our patient and staff census at the end of the field survey period. In response to special delivery letters and telephone requests, 59 of the 77 programs had replied by the end of May, 1972. A tabulation of these reports showed that the number of patients in treatment had increased by 37%. There were now 6,253 drug abusers receiving treatment in Pennsylvania. Similarly, the number of full-time staff at these 59 programs had increased by 29%—from 671 to 866. This May program census, then, indicates that the rapid expansion of drug treatment programs was continuing in the State, although caution should be exercised in accepting at face value unverified census data from drug abuse programs.

DISCUSSION

Phase I evaluation was planned as a comprehensive review of existing drug abuse treatment programs in Pennsylvania. Detailed program information was systematically obtained from all treatment facilities in the State. In this data collection procedure the on-site visit by the research team was the keystone of the evaluation design.

Our field investigation yielded voluminous epidemiological and progammatic data. While our major emphasis here is on epidemiological findings, these have been analyzed with respect to specific modalities of treatment. With regard to the programs themselves, it is pertinent in the present Phase I context to mention that we found an almost unbelievable variation in physical facilities, staffing patterns, medical service provided, equipment, administration, record-keeping procedures, and treatment ideologies.

The next step in our evaluation schema, Phase II, consists of three major undertakings: (*a*) establishing a statewide communication network and a data bank, (*b*) developing program standards and regulations for the different modalities of treatment, and (*c*) formulating a statewide coordinating plan with provisions for technical, scientific, and medical assistance to all treatment programs within the state.

The last stage in the evaluation schema, Phase III, consists of comparative outcome studies of drug-abuse treatment programs. Appropriate followup studies of former patients in the community are an indispensable part of Phase III.

REFERENCES

1. Ball, J. C., & Chambers, C. D. *The epidemiology of opiate addiction in the United States.* Springfield: Charles C. Thomas, 1970.
2. Glaser, F. B., Ball, J. C., Moffett, A. D., & Adler, F. L. The treatment of narcotic addiction in Philadelphia: Yesterday, today and tomorrow. *Philadelphia Medicine,* 67, 1971, 613–621.
3. Glasscote, R. M., Sussex, J. N., Jaffe, J. H., Ball, J. C., & Brill, L. *The treatment of drug abuse.* Washington, D.C.: Joint Information Service of the American Psychiatric Association and the National Association for Mental Health, 1972.
4. Terry, C. E., & Pellens, M. *The opium problem.* New York: Bureau of Social Hygiene, Inc., 1928.

A 48-WEEK STUDY OF METHADONE, METHADYL ACETATE, AND MINIMAL SERVICES[1]

Edward C. Senay
Illinois Drug Abuse Program and University of Chicago

Jerome H. Jaffe
Special Action Office for Drug Abuse Prevention
Executive Office of the President

Salvatore diMenza
Illinois Drug Abuse Program

and

Pierre F. Renault
University of Chicago

INTRODUCTION

A series of studies of methadyl acetate (variously called *l*-acetylmethadol [LAM] or *l*-alpha-acetylmethadol) has demonstrated tentatively that this long-lasting drug does not appear to differ from methadone in rehabilitative efficacy or safety. Interest in methadyl acetate has been generated primarily but not exclusively by its obvious potential for reducing the amount of maintenance drug that finds its way to the street.

Jaffe, Schuster, Smith, and Blachly [2] studied eight patients who received *dl*-alpha-acetylmethadol 3 times a week and placebos on alternate days, and a group of eight control patients who received daily methadone. Significant differences between these groups in terms of social performance and frequency of withdrawal symptoms were not observed. A few patients complained of anxiety; although drug factors could not be ruled out, the authors felt that nondrug factors probably offered a more parsimonious explanation of this complaint. No major side effects were encountered during the course of this 5-week study.

[1] This research was supported by U.S. Public Health Service Grant 5H17 MH 16409 and State of Illinois Mental Health Grant 2CW-2035. The authors would like to express their appreciation to Bhanwar Joshi and Young Shim Lee for their efforts in the collection and statistical analysis of the data presented.

Jaffe and Senay [3] demonstrated the practicality of repeated interchange of methadone with methadyl acetate in a study of volunteer male patients stabilized on methadone. In blind fashion they were divided into groups of subjects who continued daily methadone or who received weekday methadone and weekend methadyl acetate. Again, the performance of these groups was equivalent in terms of illicit drug use, arrest records, and clinic attendance.

In a double-blind study, Jaffe, Senay, Schuster, Renault, Smith, and diMenza [4] randomly assigned 34 chronic male heroin addicts to a methadone group or to a methadyl acetate group, and studied their progress over a 15-week period. The dose of methadyl acetate ranged from 36 to 80 mg, administered on Monday, Wednesday, and Friday of each 7-day period. A 30 mg dextromethorphan placebo was given on the remaining days. Again, no significant differences were observed in terms of narcotic-free weeks, employment status, self-reported illegal activity, or frequency of clinic attendance.

While studies conducted by the Illinois Drug Abuse Program (IDAP) failed to demonstrate differences between methadyl acetate and methadone, other workers have not corroborated these findings. Blachly, David, and Irwin [1] reported a study in which they investigated the physiological status of 21 patients taking methadyl acetate and 18 patients maintained on methadone. An analysis of EEGs from each group disclosed that 53% of all subjects had abnormal readings, but no statistically significant differences were observed between the methadone and methadyl acetate groups. Blachly also observed hyperglycemia in patients taking methadyl acetate, as well as agitation and confusion during the first 2 weeks of conversion to methadyl acetate from methadone.

Irritability was reported by three participants in a clinical trial of methadyl acetate conducted by Zaks, Fink, and Freedman [11]; however, this did not seem to affect treatment outcome. A few study subjects complained of jerkiness in the lower limbs just before sleep.

Senay and diMenza [7] reviewed in detail the side effects, advantages, and disadvantages of methadyl acetate in the treatment of heroin addiction. They noted the small number of patients studied, as well as the short duration of the projects, and concluded that additional studies are needed to explore further the safety and efficacy of methadyl acetate. The study reported below was designed to address these needs. The inclusion of a dispensary group was aimed at answering additional questions of interest.

Although methadone has been used widely, its exact role in the rehabilitation of heroin addicts remains uncertain. A critical question remains: Is the drug the treatment, or does treatment occur as a function of so-called ancillary services, or is treatment a combination effect of both?

If simple dispensation of maintenance drugs constitutes effective treatment, many more addicts can be served per treatment dollar. If methadone and methadyl acetate are sufficient to control an addict's drug-taking behavior, then the expenditure of precious resources to provide psychological counseling, psychiatric support, vocational rehabilitation, and social services would appear to be wasteful. This study was designed to compare methadone and methadyl acetate in full service clinics and at the same time to clarify the question of what constitutes treatment by comparing both groups to a group receiving methadone alone without ancillary services.

METHOD

Subjects

All male heroin addicts who applied for admission to the Illinois Drug Abuse Program between January and April, 1971, were asked to volunteer for this research project. Each potential subject was told of the effects and possible dangers of methadone and methadyl acetate, about the therapeutic regimen to be employed in each research group, and that all assignments would be on a random basis. One hundred and fifty-seven consecutive volunteers were chosen for the study and randomly assigned to study groups in the following numbers: 96 to methadone with no other services (dispensary); 30 to methadone with full services; and 31 to methadyl acetate with full services. A larger number of patients was assigned to the dispensary because it was felt that methadone dispensaries would, by design, serve more addicts than full service methadone clinics. The research dispensary was structured, therefore, with a disproportionately large patient load. All patients underwent a complete physical examination.

The Clinics and the Therapeutic Process

Two research areas were established for this study. They were contiguous and were served by the same building entrance. The dispensary area consisted of a dayroom, a nurses' station from which methadone was dispensed, and a washroom where urine specimens were monitored. A nurse who dispensed the methadone was always present in the dispensary, as was one of four counselors, all ex-addicts who had been trained by the Illinois Drug Abuse Program. Patients in the dispensary, however, were not assigned to a counselor; thus the patient–staff ratio was 90:1. The dispensary staff was instructed to keep patient contact to a minimum: If a patient sought them out they were to be friendly and enter into a conversation, but no legal, employment, psychological, recreational, or social services were to be provided.

In the dispensary area methadone was distributed in an orange drink mixture (Twist) daily between 3 PM and 6 PM, and patients were required to consume the medication in the nurse's presence. On Saturdays, patients took home one dose of methadone for use on Sunday. A patient who was employed and free of heroin use for 4 consecutive weeks would be allowed to pick up medication on Monday, Wednesday, and Friday (or Tuesday, Thursday, and Saturday).

All patients were required to give a urine specimen in the presence of a counselor every Monday and Friday. The two urines for the week were pooled and analyzed by thin-layer chromatography with hydrolysis [5]. In addition, each patient in the study was required to fill out a weekly questionnaire which dealt with drug use, employment, and illegal activity during the past week.

Transfers to other Illinois Drug Abuse Program clinics were discouraged and were undertaken only when absolutely necessary. Patients were not discharged unless their behavior severely disrupted clinic operations, frequent or prolonged absence and failure to show rehabilitative progress were not used as reasons for discharge.

The full service area consisted of a dayroom, nurses' station, two group therapy rooms, and two counselors' offices. Every patient in a full service group was requested to attend one group therapy session led by an ex-addict counselor per week. The groups did not have a static membership from week to week, meaning that a patient could, in the course of several weeks, attend group sessions conducted by different counselors and made up of different sets of group members.

The patient–staff ratio in the full service area was 20:1, and patients were encouraged to meet frequently with individually assigned counselors. Vocational rehabilitation services, legal aid, job counseling, and job placement were provided. Patients could take advantage of free outside activities, such as bowling or movies, and were free to spend as much time as they wished at the clinic, where they could play cards or socialize.

Subjects in the methadyl acetate group received medication on Monday, Wednesday, and Friday, and a 30 mg dextromethorphan placebo on intervening days. A physician who was "blind" examined the patients and recommended initial dosage levels and later changes, expressing his recommendations in milligrams of methadone. A second physician wrote the actual drug orders based upon a conversion factor of 1.2 mg of methadyl acetate for 1 mg of methadone.

RESULTS

Failure of Research Design with Respect to the Dispensary

The single most significant finding in this study was that counselors and nurses could not withhold psychological support from patients in the dispensary group. These patients received transfers and covert counseling and support when they brought their life crises and multiple nonacute needs to the attention of the staff. Both overt and covert hostility to the research design and research staff was frequently expressed by the clinical staff in weekly joint meetings. The clinical staff did an excellent job of creating a warm and accepting milieu for the full service area. Dispensary patients were sensitive to this fact, and many tried repeatedly to obtain full services; many appeared to receive encouragement from the expectation that they would receive such services when the study was completed.

Characteristics of the Three Groups

Although patients were assigned randomly, the three study groups differed with respect to age and years of addiction (Table 1). The dispensary group was significantly younger than the methadone full service group ($t = 3.38; df = 125; p < .01$) but not the methadyl acetate full service group ($t = 1.32; df = 124;$ NS).[2] In the dispensary 17.7% of the group were 21 years of age or younger; the methadyl full service group had 13.3% in this age category, while the methadone full service group had only 6.4%.

Patients in the methadone full service group had been using heroin longer than patients in the methadyl acetate group ($t = 1.85; df = 59; p < .05$) or patients in the dispensary group ($t = 3.64; df = 125; p < .01$). When age was correlated with years since first heroin use, a Pearson Product Moment correlation of .81 ($n = 155; p < .01$) was found, leading to the conclusion that the difference in age probably accounted for the difference in mean number of years of addiction.

When all three groups were tested in a single contingency test, there were no significant differences among the three groups on race, marital status, years of education, arrests in the 2 years prior to entering treatment, or employment status at the time of entry.

Outcome Measures

Although data were collected on a weekly basis, for ease of presentation most of the data are reported in terms of treatment weeks 1, 12, 24, 36, and 48. Because patients entered at different times, the term *treatment week* refers to the number of weeks a given subject had been in the study.

Clinic attendance. Table 2 presents the attendance rates of the three study groups. The values reported in the rows labeled "Present in originally assigned group" refer to the patients who were active in their respective study groups at least 1 day in the given reporting week. A cursory examination of Table 2 would lead to the conclusion that early in treatment the attendance rates for the dispensary group were lower than those observed in methadyl and methadone full service groups. This difference is especially marked in week 12, but there is a reversal in weeks 24 through 48, when the methadyl group had the lowest retention rate. These differences are not significant when the Chi-square is computed using the three groups simultaneously and when the data are dichotomized into "Present in originally assigned group" and all other status categories combined. If each group is compared with each of the others separately, however, there is a significant difference between the dispensary and

---

[2] When the age of the methadone full service group is compared to the age of the methadyl acetate full service group ($t = 1.58; df = 59;$ NS).

TABLE 1

Comparison of Characteristics of Heroin Addicts Who Were Selected
for the Three Research Groups

Variable	Group			Statistic
	Dispensary ($N = 96$)	Methadyl full service ($N = 30$)	Methadone full service ($N = 31$)	
Race (%)				$\chi^2 = 1.05; df = 4;$ $p = $ NS
White	6.3	3.3	6.5	
Black	92.7	96.7	93.5	
Other	1.0	0.0	0.0	
Age				$F = 6.08; df = 2/154;$ $p < .01$
Mean	29.3	31.7	35.2	
S. D.	8.1	8.9	8.6	
Marital status (%)				$\chi^2 = 5.29; df = 2;$ $p = $ NS
Married	44.8	36.7	64.5	
Unmarried	55.2	63.3	35.5	
Years of education				$F = .68; df = 2/153;$ $p = $ NS
Mean	11.5	11.2	11.1	
S. D.	1.4	2.6	2.3	
Number of arrests in 2 years prior to entry				$F = .19*; df = 2/152;$ $p = $ NS
Mean	1.3	1.4	1.5	
S. D.	2.6	2.6	3.8	
Years of addiction				$F = 5.02; df = 2/154;$ $p < .01$
Mean	8.2	9.9	13.5	
S. D.	7.8	8.6	8.6	
Percent employed	32.3	30.0	35.5	$\chi^2 = .21; df = 2;$ $p = $ NS

*F was based upon log $(X + 1)$ transformation because mean arrests for each group was proportional to the variance.

methadone full service groups in week 12 (χ^2 = 4.02; df = 1; $p < .05$) and between the methadone full service and methadyl full service groups in week 48 (χ^2 = 4.73; df = 1; $p < .05$). Patients falling into the category "Present in another IDAP group" were considered failures for the respective research groups because their originally assigned treatment was found to be inappropriate, necessitating a transfer to other clinics. The "Absent from all treatment" category may be the most revealing, for it indicates that half of the dispensary and the methadyl acetate groups were lost after 48 weeks, when only a quarter of the methadone group had been lost.

When the total number of weeks of attendance accumulated by each patient in his originally assigned group was calculated and averaged the following means were found: dispensary, 30.5 weeks; methadyl acetate full service, 29.7 weeks; and methadone full service, 35.3 weeks. There were no significant differences among the groups (F = 1.20; df = 2/154; p = NS).

Illicit drug use. The results of the urine analysis for the five reporting periods, showing a decrease in heroin use by all three groups, are presented in Table 3. These results are presented first in terms of the actual number of patients on whom the urine information was available (3A), and then in terms of the full original sample (3B).

Table 3A reveals that while the percentage of patients having urine specimens negative for morphine increased there was a corresponding decrease in the number of urine specimens available. Expressed in terms of remaining patients, 72.7% in the dispensary, 90.9% in the methadyl acetate full service group, and 60.0% in the methadone full service group were negative for morphine in the 48th week of treatment. When the percentage is based upon the total number of persons who originally entered treatment (Table 3B), disregarding deceased and transfers, the percentages are 33.3, 33.3, and 38.7 respectively. The latter figures can be considered a measure of the total impact of the various treatment approaches on illicit narcotic use. These values are based on the assumption that a missing urine specimen was positive, a view that seems reasonable as most of the missing urine specimens were from patients who had long gaps of absences and who had quite probably returned to heroin use. (A critique of the practice of reporting outcome statistics in terms of "remaining samples" as opposed to the original "starting samples" has been published by Maddux and Bowden [6].)

In each of the three groups, whether the statistics were based on the patients who remained in treatment or in terms of the original sample, there was a general decrease in illicit drug use but no statistically significant intergroup differences for the various weeks, although it appears that the methadone full service group exhibited greater week-to-week variability.

Dosage changes. The dispensary group accumulated a total of 2933 man weeks of treatment, during which time 88 changes were made in methadone dose levels, an average of 3 changes per 100 man weeks. The methadyl acetate full service group had 58 changes in 892 man weeks for an average of 7 changes per 100 man weeks of treatment, while the methadone full service patients

TABLE 2

Comparison of Attendance Figures of the Three Groups of Patients at 12-Week Intervals

		Treatment week				
Group	Patient status	Week 1	Week 12	Week 24	Week 36	Week 48
A: Percent in various treatment statuses						
Dispensary (N = 96)	Present in originally assigned group	96.9	68.8	65.6	62.5	45.8
	Present in another IDAP group	0.0	1.0	1.0	1.0	4.2
	Detoxified and released	0.0	0.0	0.0	0.0	0.0
	Absent from all treatment	3.1	30.2	32.3	35.4	49.0
	Deceased	0.0	0.0	1.0	1.0	1.0
Methadyl full service (N = 30)	Present in originally assigned group	96.7	73.3	56.7	50.0	36.7
	Present in another IDAP group	0.0	3.3	13.3	16.7	10.0
	Detoxified and released	0.0	0.0	0.0	0.0	0.0
	Absent from all treatment	3.3	23.3	30.0	33.3	50.0
	Deceased	0.0	0.0	0.0	0.0	3.3
Methadone full service (N = 31)	Present in originally assigned group	90.3	87.1	67.7	61.3	64.5
	Present in another IDAP group	0.0	3.2	12.9	6.5	3.2
	Detoxified and released	0.0	0.0	0.0	3.2	3.2
	Absent from all treatment	9.7	9.7	19.4	29.0	29.0
	Deceased	0.0	0.0	0.0	0.0	0.0
B: Results of statistical analyses (x^2)						
Present in originally assigned group vs. all other categories	x^2	2.47	4.02	.99	1.52	5.11
	df	2	2	2	2	2
	p	NS	NS	NS	NS	NS

TABLE 3

Results of the Urine Analysis for the Presence of Morphine Based upon Number of Specimens Available and on the Original Sample

Group	Variable	Treatment week				
		Week 1	Week 12	Week 24	Week 36	Week 48
	A: Using only specimens available					
Dispensary (N = 96)	Percent negative	28.0	60.6	65.1	61.7	72.7
	Percent available	96.9	68.8	65.6	62.5	45.8
Methadyl full service (N = 30)	Percent negative	44.8	63.6	88.2	80.0	90.9
	Percent available	96.7	73.3	56.7	50.0	36.7
Methadone full service (N = 31)	Percent negative	25.0	63.0	61.9	78.9	60.0
	Percent available	77.4	87.1	67.7	61.3	64.5
	χ^2	3.41	.09	3.82	3.15	3.39
	df	2	2	2	2	2
	p	NS	NS	NS	NS	NS
	B: Using original sample					
Dispensary (N = 96)	Percent negative	27.1	41.7	42.7	38.5	33.3
Methadyl full service (N = 30)	Percent negative	43.3	46.7	50.0	40.0	33.3
Methadone full service (N = 31)	Percent negative	19.4	54.8	41.9	48.4	38.7
	χ^2	4.59	1.67	.56	.95	.32
	df	2	2	2	2	2
	p	NS	NS	NS	NS	NS

TABLE 4

Dose Level of the Patients Who Remained Continuously in Treatment in the Original Study Group up to the Various Reporting Periods

Group	Variable	Treatment week					
		Week 1	Week 12	Week 24	Week 36	Week 48	
Dispensary	Number continuously in treatment	96	59	49	45	41
	Mean dose	41.3	44.4	49.8	51.6	51.7
	S. D.	4.6	9.8	12.0	14.1	13.9
Methadyl	Number continuously in treatment	30	24	17	10	9
full	Mean dose	57.8	66.7	79.6	87.6	93.9
service	S. D.	5.8	13.1	24.4	26.6	25.2
Methadone	Number continuously in treatment	31	26	18	12	11
full	Mean dose	40.6	51.2	57.8	70.0	70.9
service	S. D.	2.5	12.4	25.3	32.5	32.7

accumulated 92 changes for 1095 man weeks of treatment or 8 changes per 100 man weeks. There is a significant difference among the groups (χ^2 = 57.1; df = 2; $p < .01$), with the dispensary patients requesting fewer changes than patients in the full service groups. This difference probably reflects the perception of many dispensary patients that their status required low demand.

There was a significant difference in the actual doses prescribed for the patients in the three groups, both initially, in week 1 (F = 161.8; df = 2/154; $p < .01$), and at the 48th week (F = 17.5; df = 2/58; $p < .01$). When the mean dose of patients who remained continuously in treatment up to a given reporting week was calculated (Table 4), it was found that the methadyl acetate patients were being maintained at a higher dose level in the 48th week than were either the dispensary (t = 4.79; df = 9; $p < .01$) or the methadone full service patients (t = 1.76; df = 18; $p < .05$).[3] These differences were expected because methadyl acetate was prescribed at the rate of 1.2 mg of methadyl for every 1 mg of methadone. Because the methadyl acetate patients took medication 3 times a week, their total weekly dosage was much lower than that of the patients on methadone. Dispensary patients were maintained at lower methadone doses than were those in the methadone full service group, but this difference was not significant. The result of a two-tailed test for the 48th week was t = 1.90; df = 11; p = NS.

Employment. The employment rates among the three groups were not different. A comparison of employment rates of the patients present in the 36th week of treatment revealed a 36.8% increase in employment in the dispensary group, a 66.7% increase in the methadyl full service group, and no change in the methadone full service group. These values were calculated by subtracting the number of patients who were employed at entry from the number that were employed in the 36th week; the difference was then divided by the number employed at entry. The 36th week was used because by the 48th week the number of patients who were still active and on whom complete employment data were available was too small to make statistical analysis meaningful.

Table 5 presents the employment information in more detail. In the dispensary group, 36.8% of those employed at entry lost their jobs, while in the methadyl full service and methadone full service groups 100% and 50%, respectively, lost jobs. Care should be taken in the interpretation of these results because the number of patients involved is quite small. The total change in employment in each group was analyzed to determine statistical significance using the McNemar Test [10]. The changes were not significant.

Illegal activity. The measures of illegal activity available were the patients' weekly self-reports. Because the validity of self-reported criminal activity is unknown, the confidence with which the data can be interpreted is limited. Table 6 presents the percentage of patients reporting that they were not involved

---

[3] A one-tail test was used because the direction of the difference between the methadyl group and those receiving methadone was predicted at the beginning of the study.

TABLE 5

Change in Employment Status from the Time of Entry to Treatment Week 36 for Those Patients on Whom Complete Employment Information Was Available

Group	Employment status	N	%	Statistic
Dispensary		60		$\chi^2 = 1.71; df = 1; p = $ NS
	Employed at entry	19	31.7	
	Remained employed	12	63.2	
	Lost jobs	7	36.8	
	Unemployed at entry	41	68.3	
	Found employment	14	34.1	
	Remained unemployed	27	65.9	
Methadyl full service		15		$\chi^2 = 0.13; df = 1; p = $ NS
	Employed at entry	3	20.0	
	Remained employed	0	0.0	
	Lost jobs	3	100.0	
	Unemployed at entry	12	80.0	
	Found employment	5	41.7	
	Remained unemployed	7	58.3	
Methadone full service		19		$\chi^2 = 0.17; df = 1; p = $ NS
	Employed at entry	6	31.6	
	Remained employed	3	50.0	
	Lost jobs	3	50.0	
	Unemployed at entry	13	68.4	
	Found employment	3	23.1	
	Remained unemployed	10	76.9	

TABLE 6

Comparison of Self-Reported Illegal Activity Based upon the Number of Patients Available and on the Original Sample

Group	Variable	Treatment week			
		Week 1	Week 12	Week 24	Week 36
	A: Using only patients available				
Dispensary (N = 96)	Percent reporting no illegal activity	54.4	84.8	84.1	90.0
	Percent available	93.8	68.8	65.6	62.5
Methadyl full service (N = 30)	Percent reporting no illegal activity	74.1	95.5	94.1	100.0
	Percent available	90.0	73.3	56.7	50.0
Methadone full service (N = 31)	Percent reporting no illegal activity	53.6	81.5	95.2	94.7
	Percent available	90.3	87.1	67.7	61.3
	χ^2	3.55	2.17	2.56	1.91
	df	2	2	2	2
	p	NS	NS	NS	NS
	B: Using original sample				
Dispensary (N = 96)	Percent reporting no illegal activity	51.0	58.3	55.2	56.3
Methadyl full service (N = 30)	Percent reporting no illegal activity	66.7	70.0	53.3	50.0
Methadone full service (N =31)	Percent reporting no illegal activity	48.4	71.0	64.5	58.1
	χ^2	2.65	2.37	1.00	0.47
	df	2	2	2	2
	p	NS	NS	NS	NS

in any form of illegal activity, excluding drug purchases for their own use. As with the urine analysis data, the results are presented in terms of the sample remaining during the given report week and in terms of the original sample. The assumption was made, if a patient were not in treatment in a given week, that he was involved in illegal activity. The results demonstrate that the longer a patient stayed in treatment the lower his self-reported illegal activity, but at no time were these three study groups different.

An index of the rate of self-reported arrests in the research groups was determined by dividing the total number of arrests accumulated by the groups to the 36th week of treatment (the latest time period with sufficient information for analysis available) by the number of weeks for which arrest information was available. The patients in the dispensary accumulated 45 arrests for 2110 man weeks of information, or 2.1 arrests per 100 man weeks, while the methadyl full service group had 2.3 arrests per 100 man weeks (15 arrests, 661 man weeks) and the methadone full service group averaged 3.0 arrests per 100 man weeks (23 arrests, 775 man weeks). Each patient's "arrest per man week" was transformed to the log (arrests per man week + 1), and a one-way analysis of variance was performed which was not found to be significant ($F = .51; df = 2/154; p = $ NS).

Clinical Observations

Confusion, psychotic symptoms, or unpleasant subjective states were not observed in any of the study subjects. Anxiety was observed but no more often in any one group. The anxiety observed among methadyl acetate patients did not appear to have determinants different from those observed in methadone patients. In our clinical judgment drug factors did not appear to be directly implicated. Two deaths occurred in the study population: A dispensary patient committed suicide and a patient in the methadyl acetate full service group died of lung cancer.

DISCUSSION

Two reasons account for the failure to compare full services with simple dispensation. One factor was that the two study areas were contiguous. The milieu of warmth and acceptance generated in the full service area was communicated to the dispensary patients, with the result that many of these patients developed a positive feeling about their treatment experience. This was evident in their relationships in the dispensary area and had a major effect on their expectations, as substantial numbers of dispensary area patients looked forward to the end of the study when they expected to receive full services. It is important to point out that we studied full services versus minimal services, not full services versus simple dispensation as we intended at the outset of the study.

We have observed simple dispensation in clinics with minimal services. These clinics were not contiguous with full service areas, but patients in them knew about such treatment and expected to be enrolled in it after a brief interval. Although such dispensaries can function for a time, their operations tend to be problem-ridden, volatile, and frequently quite negative. Simple distribution of a drug as an extended procedure carries an unacceptably high risk of poor outcome for individual patients and for the communities in which these clinics are located. In our experience such operations are likely to be responded to negatively by community groups, and are not accepted for any extended period.

The emotional pressures generated by the dispensary situation could not be tolerated by clinical or research personnel as patients brought acute crises and multiple nonacute needs which the staff could not ignore. Clinical staff became advocates, and human needs took precedence over research needs. For example, transfers which violated the research design were effected when clinically indicated; also much covert counseling and overt support were in evidence. The clinical staff exhibited constant hostility to the issue of research and to the research staff, although they were intellectually aware of and in agreement with the merit of the research questions.

When full services are compared to minimal services the results of this study suggest that interaction affects between drug and types of services may be important. Trends in the attendance data suggest that methadone plus full services appears to be superior to both methadyl acetate plus full services and methadone plus minimal services; this difference is particularly apparent if we examine the "absent from all treatment" data (Table 2); here methadone plus full services has lost only 29% at the end of 48 weeks, while the other two groups have lost 49% (dispensary) and 50% (methadyl acetate and full service). An obvious source of variance which may play a role is dose. Methadyl acetate patients may have dropped out either because their dose was too low to suppress the appearance of the abstinence syndrome, or because for the given patient the dose was high enough to cause side effects such as irritability or anxiety.

Previous works [8, 9] describe a theory which attributes the success of methadone maintenance to the combination of methadone plus a positive institutional transference. The results of the present study, particularly considering the relative success of the methadone plus minimal services group (dispensary), seem to provide further support to this theory: because methadone plus positive institutional transference can define treatment it does not necessarily follow that this contribution should define treatment. Clearly this minimal combination can also turn into an ugly community problem. Provision of full service improves upon the result of the base combination and provides a minimal precondition for community acceptance. We contend that without community acceptance and participation the gains achieved by the medical model of methadone maintenance will be rapidly dissipated as the familiar forces of poverty, joblessness, and disenfranchisement take effect.

The comparison of methadone and methadyl acetate was the second major focus of this study. The outstanding finding in this respect is the trend suggesting that methadone has greater holding power than methadyl acetate. The generalizability of our findings in this the longest controlled study of methadyl acetate and methadone reported to date by the Illinois Drug Abuse Program is limited by differences among study groups which result from random assignment. Methadone full service patients in comparison to methadyl acetate full service patients were older, more likely to be married, and had used heroin for a longer period of time (Table 1). Such older, married, more seasoned addicts may tend to have greater motivation for change and therefore have a greater tendency to stay in treatment; therefore, nondrug factors could account for differences observed.

But when attendance data for all three groups are compared it appears that drug factors do play a role and that methadone may have a greater power than methadyl acetate to hold patients in clinics. The dispensary group was younger, although the difference was not statistically significant, than the methadyl acetate group but comparable to it in all other respects. The attendance of the dispensary group was consistently equal to or better than that observed in the methadyl acetate full service group despite the fact that only minimal services accompanied the drug. The differences reasonably can be attributed to the difference in drugs. Because methadone alone is roughly equivalent to methadyl acetate plus full services in holding power, and because methadone plus full services is better than either, we tentatively conclude that methadone has greater holding power than methadyl acetate. We recognize that further research is needed before a definitive statement can be made in this regard.

We did not observe that patients were able to detect which drug they were receiving. We also did not observe the side effects reported by Blachly et al. [1] and by Zaks et al. [11]. Gross differences in safety between methadone and methadyl acetate were not observed in this study.

SUMMARY

Difficulties in carrying out the design of this study weaken the generalizability of the findings. In effect we studied full services versus minimal services. Interactions between drugs and types of services were important. Methadone plus full services appeared to be superior to methadyl acetate plus full services or methadone plus minimal services. Results of this appear to confirm trends noted in prior studes [2, 4], suggesting that methadone has a greater holding power than methadyl acetate. But because random assignment resulted in sufficient dissimilarities between study groups more research is needed before we can have confidence than any difference exists. Methadyl acetate did not appear to differ from methadone in safety or subjective effects in the course of this study.

REFERENCES

1. Blachly, P. H., David, N. A., & Irwin, S. *l*-Alpha-acetylmethadol (LAM): Comparison of laboratory findings, electroencephalograms, and Cornell Medical Index of patients

stabilized on LAM with those on methadone. *Fourth National Conference on Methadone Treatment Proceedings,* San Francisco, Jan. 8-10, 1972. New York: National Association for the Prevention of Addiction to Narcotics, 203-206, 1972.

2. Jaffe, J. H., Schuster, C. R., Smith, B. B., & Blachly, P. H. Comparison of acetyl-methadol and methadone in the treatment of long-term heroin users. *JAMA,* 211, 1834-1836, 1970.

3. Jaffe, J. H., & Senay, E. C. Methadone and *l*-methadyl acetate: Use in management of narcotics addicts. *JAMA,* 216, 1303-1305, 1971.

4. Jaffe, J. H., Senay, E. C., Schuster, C. R., Renault, P. F., Smith, B. B., & diMenza, S. Methadyl acetate vs. methadone: A double-blind study in heroin users. *JAMA,* 222, 437-442, 1972.

5. Kaistha, K. K., & Jaffe, J. H. Extraction techniques for narcotics, barbiturates, and central nervous system stimulants in a drug abuse urine screening program. *Journal of Chromatography,* 60, 83-94, 1971.

6. Maddux, J. F., & Bowden, C. L. Critique of success with methadone maintenance. *American Journal of Psychiatry,* 129, 440-446, 1972.

7. Senay, E. C., & diMenza, S. Methadyl acetate in treatment of heroin addiction: A review. Proceedings, National Research Council, May, 1972. Ann Arbor, Michigan. In press.

8. Senay, E. C., & Wright, M. Critique of theories of methadone use. Paper presented at the Second International Symposium on Drug Abuse, Jerusalem, 1972.

9. Senay, E. C., & Wright, M. The human needs approach to the treatment of drug dependence. Paper presented at the International Council on Alcoholism and Addiction, Amsterdam, 1972.

10. Siegel, S. *Nonparametric statistics for the behavioral sciences.* New York: McGraw-Hill, 1956.

11. Zaks, A., Fink, M., & Freedman, A. M. *l*-Alpha-acetylmethadol in maintenance treatment of opiate dependence. *Fourth National Conference on Methadone Treatment Proceedings,* San Francisco, Jan. 8-10, 1972. New York: National Association for the Prevention of Addiction to Narcotics, 207-210, 1972.

QUESTIONS IN CYCLAZOCINE
THERAPY OF OPIATE DEPENDENCE[1]

Max Fink
State University of New York—Stony Brook

In the absence of a specific prophylaxis for opiate dependence, and with the likelihood that drug use will remain one of the nation's principal avocations, fostered by government, industry, and the communication media, there is a need to find treatment strategies that may help the individual victim of addiction and dependence. From an organismic point of view, three hypotheses of the mode of dependence development have led to three therapeutic tactics:

1. The view that individual psychosocial development is a critical factor and can be mobilized by will power, group identification, group process, and social manipulation has led to nonpharmacologic, therapeutic communities like Phoenix Houses.

2. The view that drug abuse is irremedial, with accompanying induced metabolic defects justifying the replacement of illicit, short-acting opiates by licit, long-acting formulations, has led to an extensive federal, state, and private methadone delivery network.

3. The view that conditioning aspects contribute heavily to the recidivism after withdrawal from opiates and that some use may be made of extinction processes has led to the testing of narcotic antagonists and the deconditioning paradigm [12, 13, 17].

Others have elaborated the conditions favorable for drug-free therapeutic communities and have supported the development of a large opiate delivery

[1] The work reported here was done at the New York Medical College and the Metropolitan Hospital Mental Health Center, 1966–1972; aided by MH 19476 from the National Institute of Mental Health and by a contract with the New York State Narcotic Addiction Control Commission.

system. In our laboratories, we have examined these approaches, and found both their long-term merit and their short-term challenge uninspiring and unrewarding. With regard to methadone, for example, the question "After methadone, what?" troubles us; and each time we are seduced by political, social, or financial pressures to expand our present methadone and levomethadyl comparison sample to a larger delivery and maintenance system, we face the additional question "If not now, when?" as the challenge for both the patient and ourselves. We have focused our efforts on examining the narcotic antagonists.

The history of the use of extinction methods based on the specific narcotic antagonists has been presented elsewhere [1], and its logic has been elaborated by Martin [13] and Wikler [17]. While a favorable climate for extinction and deconditioning may be provided by intensive rehabilitation and group processes, these methods are expensive and time-consuming. Thus, the potential of agents that blocked the euphoria of each administration of opiates was examined. Methadone was considered, for tolerance to high doses of methadone "blocks" the euphoria of the usual street doses of opiates by cross-tolerance. But methadone produces its own dependence, and a nonaddicting, blocking agent was sought, and found in cyclazocine. Cyclazocine is a specific narcotic antagonist with a low dependence potential and a long duration of action. Cyclazocine, however, exhibits agonistic features, and the early studies were focused on its clinical pharmacology [1, 2, 5, 7, 8, 9, 10, 12]. (Reports of unpleasant secondary effects elicited when induction procedures were still primitive are often quoted as objections to the use of cyclazocine.) Other antagonists have received some study, such as naloxone [6, 19], naloxone pamoate, and high-dose cyclazocine [16]. The studies of cyclazocine provide answers to the pharmacologic questions of dosage, route, rate of induction, side effects, and their management with naloxone. A few studies have inquired into the personality predictors for the successful use of cyclazocine [14], its antidepressant effects, and its neurophysiologic characteristics [2].

Because of the difficulties in the use of cyclazocine described by other workers, it may be useful to review our present procedures and recent experience.

METHODS

In our laboratories, we have examined opiate addicts who volunteer for admission to an inpatient treatment center in a municipal hospital in the East Harlem section of New York City. The population of this community is very low-income, predominantly black and Puerto Rican, with low educational levels and a high incidence of unemployment and public assistance. They ranged in age from 17 to 54 with a mean of 26 years, and their duration of opiate addiction was from 2 to 30 years.

On admission to a study ward, methadone is given twice daily in decreasing amounts for detoxification. Usually within 4 to 7 days the subject is drug-free, and a period of observation without drugs allows medical and laboratory examinations before induction with an antagonist.

Cyclazocine has been studied since 1966. The first studies reported inductions and maintenance programs on 4 mg cyclazocine [12].

Induction

We first attempted to develop an induction schedule which would minimize dysphoria. The dosage of cyclazocine was gradually increased in groups of patients to 4.0 mg/day in 10, 15, 20, 30, and 40 days. The more rapid the induction schedule, the higher the incidence of complaints of somnolence, headache, irritability, and "fuzzy thinking." We found the 20- to 40-day induction periods to be well tolerated without these symptoms [4, 5, 7, 8]. We settled on the 20-day schedule and used this schedule until reports that naloxone antagonized the agonistic effects of cyclazocine led us to reduce the induction schedule [10]. We tested patients with increments of 1.0 mg cyclazocine a day until a 4.0 mg single dose was reached in 4 days. Initially, we gave patients 0.5-1.0 gm oral naloxone only when they complained of unpleasant symptoms, and found that naloxone was necessary in only a few patients. Of 60 patients inducted on this rapid schedule, less than one-third requested naloxone, usually during the 3rd-6th days [15].

Fifty additional subjects have since been inducted by this rapid method with no subjects failing to complete the induction schedule. Secondary effects, when present, gradually subside within 5-15 days.

Dosage

We and others found 4.0 mg/day to be an effective dose [7, 8]. Following our successful extension of the duration of action of naloxone by massive daily dosages, Resnick in our laboratories used this paradigm for cyclazocine and increased its dosage to 20 mg/day [16]. Dosages were increased in increments of 0.5 mg every 3 to 5 days to 10 mg/day; thereafter by increments of 1.0 mg/week to 20 mg. While these increments were accompanied by transient secondary effects of light-headedness and sedation, tolerance developed rapidly, and the higher doses have been well sustained.

Heroin Challenges

Because we were interested in measuring the efficacy and duration of antagonism of cyclazocine to opiates, we developed the "heroin challenge" as an index of blockade. Subjective response to selected questions of the morphine scale of the NIMH Addiction Research Center Inventory, pupillary size, respiratory rate, and electroencephalographic measures are used as indices of responses [18].

During the induction phase, narcotic blocking activity of cyclazocine is discussed in individual and group therapy sessions with all the resident addicts.

They are offered an opportunity for an intravenous injection of heroin in the laboratory when they are receiving a full daily dose of cyclazocine. We have determined that 25 mg heroin/2 cc saline/2 minutes elicits both the behavioral effects and EEG changes in patients 7–10 days after a final dose of methadone during the detoxification schedule, when they are "clean."

We challenged patients 24 hours after single daily doses of 4.0 mg cyclazocine. Two-thirds experienced no clinical effects and one-third exhibited euphoria. The dose of these patients was raised to 6.0 mg, and usually there was no response to a second heroin challenge 24 hours after the higher dose of cyclazocine [4, 5].

In patients challenged with 25 mg heroin after the higher doses of cyclazocine, we have observed an extension of blockade to 48 hours after 10 mg, and to 72 hours after the 20 mg dose [16].

Supportive Therapies and Aftercare

Psychotherapy, education and job counseling, social casework, and welfare assistance are important aspects of the treatment process. In a population of lower-class indigent patients we have been impressed that their inadequate educational and work experience prejudices their discharge to the community. To assist their readjustment as well as to intensify their engagement to therapy, we enroll patients in therapeutic groups, job counseling, re-education, and family and marital guidance. Following the experimental deconditioning paradigms from animal psychology, we have accepted careful handling, reduction of interpersonal anxiety, and an inviting clinical setting as particularly beneficial aspects of antagonist therapy.

Patients are able to interrupt a cyclazocine schedule without symptoms of withdrawal. On the day that a 4.0 or 5.0 mg cyclazocine dose is not taken, they are able to experience the euphoric and sedative effects of heroin. At the higher doses, a proportionately longer period must elapse before heroin effects can be experienced. But by reinstituting cyclazocine, physiologic dependence is often deterred.

Patients receiving cyclazocine demonstrate changes in their daily behavior. Drug-seeking behavior decreases, criminality declines, and interest in vocational activities is enhanced. Social activities and leisure time spent with nonaddicts are increased. But the use of alcohol, marijuana, and other drugs is not affected; their use, if previously present, continues. Contrary to expectation, patients do not turn to other drugs or to alcohol *de novo*.

After discharge, patients are asked to attend the clinic for medication as frequently as consistent with their social and personal circumstances, such as their job, the distance they live from the hospital, and our assessment of clinical improvement. The alliance of a reliable family member in monitoring drug intake has been particularly helpful. Such supervision has been invaluable, both to decrease the frequency of clinic visits and because failure to take medication is interpreted as an announcement that illicit drug use is planned or anticipated, and family or professional intervention can be encouraged. The frequency of clinic visits ranges from daily to once every 2 weeks. The patients are seen by a therapist as their interest and clinical needs require and are encouraged to call upon a social worker, teacher, or rehabilitation counselor.

Tolerance to the antinarcotic activity of cyclazocine has not been observed. Patients receiving a heroin challenge 2 years after their induction period show as much blockade to heroin as when the challenge was given at the end of induction.

RESULTS

We have inducted more than 300 patients to cyclazocine since 1967. Of our early inductions, few remain—in part because we were exploring the clinical pharmacology, and in part because we failed to appreciate the importance of supportive services. In the summary published at the end of 1971, we noted that of 59 new patients inducted in 1969 and 1970, 37 remained in treatment and 22 had discontinued [15]. A recent assessment (October 1972) showed that selecting patients on the basis of their preference for cyclazocine treatment has yielded a favorable outcome in more than 50% of the subjects.

We find that withdrawal from cyclazocine can be accomplished easily and without difficulty. Thus far, we have waited for patients to make this request rather than suggesting it to them. Every patient who elected to withdraw from cyclazocine with our consent has either remained drug free or requested to be reinducted on cyclazocine because he reported drug-seeking behavior to persist. Twenty-one patients are currently withdrawn from cyclazocine and are drug free (October 1972). Eleven of these subjects had been previously withdrawn and then requested reinduction. Their mean time on cyclazocine is 28.7 months (range 8 to 64 months) and their mean time without cyclazocine is 10 months (range 1 month to 20 months) [16].

In these same patient populations, we have studied naloxone, l-cyclazocine, and naloxone pamoate. None provides blockade of longer duration than cyclazocine, and more extensive studies have not been undertaken with these compounds.

DISCUSSION

Our experience in developing a delivery system for cyclazocine and the associated therapies for a therapeutic modality continues to impress us that this treatment is feasible, safe, and often successful. The principal limitation to its use remains the duration of action for daily administration; at the least, once every other day is necessary. This limitation motivates the search for physical means to extend its duration and for other compounds with an inherently longer duration of activity. We have discontinued our studies of naloxone, naloxone pamoate, and the levo-isomer of cyclazocine. We have eschewed studies of BC-2605 since its pharmacology does not suggest superiority to cyclazocine. We look forward to studies of oral naltrexone and diprenorphine directed to providing an antagonist with a greater duration of action and perhaps an easier induction than that of cyclazocine.

The issue today, however, is not the clinical study of the "drug of the month" but an adequate examination of the deconditioning hypothesis. We have provided sufficient evidence of the safety and efficacy of cyclazocine as an antagonist, but we do not know what other aspects are essential for the therapeutic process.

What psychotherapeutic and retraining procedures are essential for extinction of dependence and drug-seeking behavior?

Do challenges with intraveous opiates enhance this process, and if so, at what frequency and under what conditions? Or do exposures to opiates, even without euphoria and evidence of CNS effects, still stimulate the dependence process and extend the liability for recidivism?

If cyclazocine is useful, can we extend its duration of action even further by doses higher than 20 mg every other day? At what cost? (Others have experimented with low, essentially ineffective blocking doses of naloxone and reported therapeutic failure, suggesting that effective blockade may indeed be essential to the therapeutic process.)

In what ways does a deconditioning regimen using a narcotic antagonist differ from that based on a drug-free approach (as in Phoenix House)? Such a comparison would provide some data on the ingredients essential for the deconditioning process.

Meanwhile, the nation is embarked on a large-scale methadone experiment. With the demand for daily dosages, seepage of illicit methadone is an increasing reality. Reports that acetylmethadols extend the duration of opiate action led to the testing of two formulations, methadyl acetate and levomethadyl. Methadyl acetate, as reported by Senay, Jaffe, and Blachly (see Senay, et al., this volume), is effective for 48 to 72 hours with some agonistic side effects. In our studies of levomethadyl, we observed a safe and effective schedule with delivery 3 times a week for doses of 70-90 mg [3, 11, 20]. Perhaps, as an interim measure, the administrative delays and dependence on animal toxicology inherent in the testing of new drugs could be relieved sufficiently to allow a more rapid testing of the substitution of levomethadyl for methadone in man—particularly in anticipation of the backlash now promised as more and more practitioners and local governments embark on their individual methadone delivery systems with the attendant increased risks of seepage and toxicity. Having contributed to the narcotic antagonist studies of the past 7 years, I have become increasingly concerned that we have, unwittingly perhaps, encouraged powerful political forces to deliver therapies that have been inadequately tested and whose theoretic foundations have been poorly explored. Perhaps we can begin to earn absolution by a more rapid testing of levomethadyl in man [3].

For the narcotic antagonists, the issues of extinction and the deconditioning hypothesis still remain. Perhaps, at a similar symposium a few years hence, a satisfactory test of this hypothesis will be discussed.

REFERENCES

1. Fink, M. Narcotic antagonists in opiate dependence. *Science*, 159, 1005–1006, 1970.
2. Fink, M. Treatment and prevention of opiate dependence with narcotic antagonists. *Contemp. drug problems*, 1, 245–262, 1972.
3. Fink, M. Levomethadyl (LAAM): A long-acting substitute for methadone in maintenance therapy of opiate dependence. In J. Masserman (Ed.), *Current psychiatric therapies.* New York: Grune & Stratton, in press.
4. Fink, M., & Freedman, A. M. Antagonists in the treatment of opiate dependence. In R. V. Phillipson (Ed.), *Modern trends in combatting drug dependence and alcoholism.* London: Butterworth, 1970.
5. Fink, M., Freedman, A. M., Zaks, A., Sharoff, R. L., & Resnick, R. B. Narcotic antagonists and substitutes in opiate dependence. In A. Cerletti & F. J. Bove (Eds.), *The present status of psychotropic drugs.* Excerpta Medica, Amsterdam, pp. 428–431, 1969.
6. Fink, M., Zaks, A., Sharoff, R. L., Mora, A., Bruner, A., Levit, S., & Freedman, A. M. Naloxone in heroin dependence. *Clin. Pharm. Therap.*, 9, 568–577, 1968.
7. Freedman, A. M., Fink, M., Sharoff, R. L., & Zaks, A. Cyclazocine and methadone in narcotic addiction. *JAMA*, 202, 191–194, 1967.
8. Freedman, A. M., Fink, M., Sharoff, R. L., & Zaks, A. Clinical studies of cyclazocine in the treatment of narcotic addiction. *Amer. J. Psychiat.*, 124, 1499–1504, 1968.
9. Jaffe, J. H., & Brill, L. Cyclazocine, a long acting narcotic antagonist: Its voluntary acceptance as a treatment modality by narcotic abusers. *Int. J. Addiction*, 1, 99–123, 1966.
10. Jasinski, D. R., Martin, W. R., & Haertzen, C. A. The human pharmacology and abuse potential of *N*-allylnoroxymorphone (naloxone). *J. Pharmacol. Exp. Therap.*, 157, 420–426, 1967.
11. Levine, R., Zaks, A., Fink, M., & Freedman, A. M. Levomethadyl: Prolonged duration of opioid effects, including cross tolerance to heroin, in Man. *J.A.M.A.* (in press).
12. Martin, W. R., Gorodetzky, C. W., & McClane, T. K. An experimental study in the treatment of narcotic addicts with cyclazocine. *Clin. Pharm. Therap.*, 7, 455–465, 1966.
13. Martin, W. R. Opioid antagonists. *Pharmacol. Rev.*, 19, 463–521, 1967.
14. Resnick, R. B., Fink, M., & Freedman, A. M. A cyclazocine typology in opiate dependence. *Amer. J. Psychiat.*, 126, 1256–1260, 1970.
15. Resnick, R. B., Fink, M., & Freedman, A. M. Cyclazocine therapy of opiate dependence— A progress report. *Compr. Psychiat.*, 12, 491–502, 1971.
16. Resnick, R. B., Fink, M., & Freedman, A. M. High-dose cyclazocine therapy of opiate dependence. In preparation.
17. Wikler, A. Conditioning factors in opiate addiction and relapse. In D. M. Wilner & G. G. Kassebaum (Eds.), *Narcotics.* New York: McGraw-Hill, 1965.
18. Zaks, A., Bruner, A., Fink, M., & Freedman, A. M. Intravenous diacetylmorphine (heroin) in studies of opiate dependence. *Dis. Nerv. Syst. (Suppl.)*, 30, 89–92, 1969.
19. Zaks, A., Jones, T., Fink, M., & Freedman, A. M. Treatment of opiate dependence with high dose oral naloxone. *JAMA*, 215, 2108–2110, 1971.
20. Zaks, A., Fink, M., & Freedman, A. M. Levomethadyl in maintenance treatment of opiate dependence. *JAMA*, 220, 811–813, 1972.

CLINICAL EXPERIENCES WITH NARCOTIC ANTAGONISTS[1]

Herbert D. Kleber
Connecticut Mental Health Center

and

Yale University School of Medicine

The bright promises of the 1960s in the treatment of narcotic addiction were the therapeutic community as pioneered by Synanon and Daytop Village, and methadone maintenance as pioneered by Drs. Dole and Nyswander. These programs were so promising that they were widely copied throughout the country, the proponents of each proclaiming them to be the main answer to addiction. In the past few years the deficits in both approaches have become increasingly apparent [4, 7, 8], and the search has intensified for still newer methods. Narcotic antagonists are being hailed as one such answer even though the state of their technological development currently makes it difficult to accurately gauge their full potential. The Drug Dependence Unit (DDU) of the Connecticut Mental Health Center in New Haven has been working with narcotic antagonists since February 1970; as we describe here the various therapeutic approaches we have used with these agents, some advantages as well as some difficulties of the antagonists will become apparent.

ENTRANCE INTO PROGRAM

The modalities in which narcotic antagonists are used are part of the overall clinical program of the Drug Dependence Unit. The Unit itself encompasses, in

[1] This work was supported by Public Health Service grant MH-16356 from the National Institute of Mental Health and by Public Health Service contract HSM-42-72-211 from the National Institute of Mental Health.

Dr. Ralph Jacobsen of Endo Laboratories, Garden City, New York, supplied the naloxone for this study and was of help throughout.

addition to these, several other programs: a short-term residential treatment center, a long-term residential treatment center, a methadone maintenance program, outpatient groups, a day hospital, and various screening and outreach functions. The program has been in existence since 1968 [6]. All individuals seeking therapy at any of the DDU programs come to the screening component for determination of which program they will go into. They are initially interviewed by the full-time screening staff and then are seen by a committee made up of one representative from each of the clinical programs. This committee determines the eventual assignment of the patient, a decision based on such factors as the individual's drug history, social stability, psychological problems, and legal pressure. The individual's own preference is also given some weight, although this is not the conclusive factor.

To be admitted to the program in which naloxone is used, individuals must be aged 14–24 (under 18, signed permission from a parent or guardian is also required) and have used heroin at least 3 months. Excluded are individuals with active liver disease, acute psychotic reactions, and severe mixed addictions. To be admitted to the cyclazocine program, individuals must be at least 18 and have used heroin at least 2 years. Similar exclusions hold as with the naloxone program.

NALOXONE

Induction

Prior to beginning on naloxone, the patient has to be narcotic-free for at least 3–5 days. Initially this was accomplished by hospitalizing the heroin addict and withdrawing him via methadone substitution and withdrawal. He was kept as an inpatient for 5–7 days after the last dose of methadone and then discharged to begin naloxone. As we gained more experience with the drug and as addicts in the New Haven area also learned more about it, we were comfortable having both the detoxification and waiting period occur on an outpatient basis with very frequent urine monitoring. When necessary, however, inpatient detoxification remains available and is used, depending on the staff assessment of the patient's particular situation.

On the first naloxone day, the patient is given 100 mg at approximately 9:30 AM. He is then checked carefully for the presence of any side effects that might indicate serious withdrawal. If nothing untoward has happened, an additional 100 mg is given late in the afternoon. The naloxone is then increased by 100 mg daily until a dose of 800 mg a day is reached.

The final dosage used, 800 mg, is considered sufficient to block 50 mg of heroin for 18 hours [2, 12]. This dosage was used initially because of our desire to keep the dose as low as possible until further research had been done at higher dose levels. When this research was later done, we decided to continue with the 800 mg level both because it had been working satisfactorily from a clinical point of view and because the supply of naloxone obtainable was very limited.

Increasing the dose to 3,000 mg to provide a 24-hour blockade would have necessitated decreasing the number of patients treated by one-half to two-thirds. The naloxone is given in 200 mg tablets, with careful attention by the nursing staff to prevent their being palmed or "cheeked." The liquid form has been tried but was too unpalatable.

Routine Laboratory Procedures

1. Prior to treatment
   a. Complete physical examination
   b. CBC and differential
   c. Platelet count
   d. Liver battery
   e. Serology
   f. Urinalysis
   g. Chest X-ray
2. At 3 to 6 months
   a. CBC and differential
   b. Platelet count
   c. Liver battery
   d. Urinalysis
3. Urine examinations for narcotics, quinine, cocaine, and amphetamines are done on a supervised basis on a random schedule in which an examination is done at least once a week. Barbiturates are checked for approximately once a month unless clinical indications suggest more frequent testing.

Naloxone with a Traditionally Structured Day Program—February 1970 to Fall of 1971

Prior to our obtaining naloxone the DDU offered an additional alternative to the usual therapeutic community or methadone maintenance possibilities. This was a day treatment abstinence program, from 9 to 4, five days a week, for individuals in the 14 to 24 age range. When naloxone became available in January of 1970 it was incorporated into this program. Because of space and staff limitations the program size had to be kept to 12 to 15 individuals at any one time. Staff consisted of a mental health professional (social worker) and ex-addicts.

The program was structured on a seven-step basis, with steps reflecting changes in the patient's self-perception, attitudes toward others, drug use, ability to handle social and educational situations, and willingness to get involved in community work related to drug prevention. These changes were to be brought about in more or less conventionally run therapy groups and intensive group work focused on reality situations. In addition, the program used various "alternative high" approaches, both to introduce patients to methods of feeling good nonchemically and as a way of holding them in treatment for the short run while the longer-range effects of more conventional therapy could take hold.

Examples of "alternative highs" were a sailing program, a drama group, yoga, and use of closed circuit TV equipment. In the sailing program a large sailboat that had been donated to the DDU was scraped down and overhauled by the members, who then learned how to sail and spent some enjoyable hours on Long Island Sound. In the drama activity, individuals developed their own play so successfully that they presented numerous performances for community groups, some of which paid them for the presentation. Using a small grant from the Connecticut Commission on the Arts, we were able to obtain a part-time professional director to work with the drama group. In addition to these activities, the members set up a TV workshop with the television equipment where they learned how to operate the equipment, make TV films, and use them in various contexts.

The naloxone part of the program was reasonably successful. Patient acceptance of the drug was good, there were no serious side effects, and the patients that remained in treatment did not go to alternative drugs to continue to get a high. The other part of the program, however, was not nearly so successful. In spite of the large investment of money, time, and staff energy, the program appeared chronically disorganized, the life styles of many of the participants did not seem to change, and the split rate approached 70%.

Naloxone with a Modified Concept Day Program— December 1971 to December 1972

Because of the above problems, in the late fall of 1971 the program was completely reorganized. Individuals who were graduates of our long-term residential program, Daytop, were brought in to run the program. The day-by-day organization and ideology were changed, reflecting a modified concept with a heavy emphasis additionally on educational and vocational preparation. The "alternative high" approach was dropped. Use of the antagonist, naloxone, remained the same, with individuals receiving it once a day at an 800 mg dosage. Space was found to increase the number of day patients at any one time from 15 up to 45. With these changes the split rate gradually dropped by two-thirds.

During an average week, the program member spends time in group therapy (primarily the confrontation type), seminars, educational classes, work assignments around the facility, and recreational activities. The day hospital approach in which the individual has to deal with an outside life every evening and weekend makes it possible each day to take up issues relating to what is going on with his family, his friends, and drug-taking temptations on the street. These issues are dealt with by the therapeutic structure of the program while the naloxone provides a blockade against the temptations to use narcotic drugs. Approximately once a month a marathon group is held from Friday evening till Sunday evening.

The naloxone is typically given for 4 months, with the individual remaining in the day program an additional 2 to 3 months in the same therapeutic structure but without a blockading agent. Following successful completion of these phases, the individual moves to an evening phase, working or going to school during the day and coming in for one or two evening groups. The time in this phase is open-ended, depending upon the individual's continued progress in both psychological and social rehabilitation.

In retrospect, the success of the reorganized day program may have had less to do with the changed content of the program than with the tight organizational and disciplinary structure and the therapeutic community ideology that the Daytop graduates brought to the program. The naloxone use remained a constant.

During the 12 months beginning December 1971, 82 patients were admitted to the day program. The patients were predominantly male (70%) and almost evenly divided racially (54% white, 44% black, 2% Spanish-speaking). The median age range was 19–21 and median years of heroin use was 2–3 years. Most (69%) had some sort of legal pressure, which included awaiting trial, probation, or parole. Median years of completed schooling was 11. (Table 1)

At the end of the 12-month period, the majority of the patients were still in treatment (70%) although less than half still needed to be on the antagonist. A small number (11%) had successfully completed both the day and out-patient phases of treatment, while a somewhat larger number (18%) had left, two-thirds on their own and one-third on the program's decision. (Table 2) Use of heroin during the year was minimal (less than 2% of urines), as was use of other drugs detectable by the urine examinations (less than 4% of urines). The relative lack

TABLE 1

Characteristics of Patients Admitted to Program
December 1971–December 1972

N = 82	Percent	*N* = 82	Percent
Sex:		Heroin use:	
Male	70	1 year or less	29
Female	30	2–3 years	36
		4–5 years	29
Race:		6 years or more	6
Black	44		
Spanish	2	Legal pressure:	
White	54	No	31
		Yes	69
Age:			
18 or less	26	Schooling completed:	
19–21	36	10 years or less	34
22–24	28	11 years	19
25 or more	9	12 years	34
		13 years or more	13

TABLE 2

Status of Patients
December 1972

$N = 82$	Percent
Graduated from program	11
Still in treatment	70
On naloxone	43
Post-naloxone phase	22
Residential treatment	34
Out of treatment	18
Left by own decision	61
Asked to leave	39

of challenges to the blockading effect appears to reflect the program's strict attitude toward drug use and perhaps also the myth—which sprang up early in the program among the members—that use of narcotics after a naloxone dose makes one sick. Although persistently denied by staff, this belief apparently continues to be held among patients.

Side Effects

The side effects of naloxone that members have complained of tend to occur during the first few weeks of treatment, do not last, and, although they are at times annoying, have not presented a problem regarding the continuation of patients in treatment. Such effects are principally nausea, anorexia, sleepiness or insomnia, and difficulty in concentrating. To avoid overemphasizing the role of medication or of side effects and to decrease contagiousness of symptoms, early in our use of naloxone we developed the practice of discouraging discussion of any side effects during the group therapy sessions. Any patient having problems of any kind with the naloxone is to discuss them with either the program nurse or the physician. Once this rule was instituted, the number of complaints about the medication dropped sharply and has remained low. Four of the over 140 patients who have been on naloxone have had to be discontinued for symptoms that may have been drug related—one for severe erythema multiforme and three for gastrointestinal symptoms [9]. There have been no untoward laboratory findings to date. No withdrawal effects have been noted when the naloxone was halted.

CYCLAZOCINE

In the fall of 1972 the DDU began to use an additional narcotic antagonist, cyclazocine. Our experiences with naloxone had favorably predisposed us toward antagonists, and we were looking for an agent that would provide a longer duration of action. We hoped to use cyclazocine in a population that either did not need or would be unwilling to enter the all-day program that we used with naloxone. With the inherently longer blockade that cyclazocine provided [3], we hoped to be able to attract individuals who needed some blockading effect, were uninterested in or unsuitable for methadone, and could be expected, after a relatively short time, to be involved in some alternate all-day activities, such as school or work. The cyclazocine program, therefore, is used as a low-intervention model in which the individual comes in daily for his cyclazocine and two evenings a week for group therapy. After a given time the patient is expected to be working or in school during the day; if he is not, an evaluation is made of the possible need for more intense interventions, such as the day or residential programs. Cyclazocine is used at a maintenance dose of 4 mg, with induction taking place very slowly at a rate of 0.2 mg a day.

Our first 10 patients were inducted on a complete inpatient basis to gain experience as far as the drug and any possible side effects were concerned. Since then we have moved to outpatient induction using the same prior detoxification methods described earlier under induction to naloxone. As with naloxone, we have not found outpatient induction to present any great difficulties. Although we have used cyclazocine only for approximately 4 months, we have found that many of the side effects reported in the cyclazocine literature have not been a problem with the slow induction method [2]. Furthermore, when annoying side effects occur they tend to be easily treated by the temporary use of naloxone, 200-500 mg orally once daily [1, 5]. The side effects we have encountered have been during the induction phase and have not lasted. The predominant ones are drowsiness, constipation, and a feeling of dizziness in some cases and of being high or "spaced" in other cases. Other occasional side effects have included nausea and racing thoughts. Only one patient has had to give up the cyclazocine because of side effects, and it is not clear whether the individual's psychological state was more relevant than the side effects in causing discontinuation. In general, cyclazocine has appeared to be tolerated well from the attitudinal point of view by the members of the program. To date, however, we do not have sufficient experience to state whether the relatively low psychological intervention combined with the cyclazocine will have a substantive effect in helping individuals remain off narcotic drugs and changing their life styles.

DISCUSSION AND CONCLUSIONS

The structure of all the DDU programs is one that both discourages and is intolerant of continued illegal drug use [6]. This is more possible in a relatively small city such as New Haven, where staff and patients become quickly aware of patients' activities outside of program hours, than it would be in a larger city. This circumstance and the quality of therapeutic intervention have resulted in relatively little testing of the antagonist blockade. Such lack of challenges makes it unlikely that the program provides any direct test of the Wikler hypothesis [10, 11] concerning the use of narcotic antagonists in the extinction of the conditioned behavior of addiction. However, it is possible that some sort of extinction is going on, not to the drug effects per se or to the needle ritual but to the circumstances surrounding the obtaining and use of drugs. This may occur since the patients are back in their communities on evenings and weekends, at times inevitably in those environs where they obtained or used drugs. Continued abstinence in such situations could be associated with eventual extinction of drug-seeking behavior.

Our experience further suggests that often antagonists alone are not sufficient to keep patients in treatment long enough for change to take place. Our initial experiences with naloxone demonstrated that where the therapeutic intervention is not considered by the patients to meet their needs, they vote with their feet and leave the program. On the other hand, we are convinced on the basis of our clinical experience with addicts over the past 4½ years that the treatment intervention without the antagonists would yield equally dismal results. That is, our experience had indicated that heroin addicts treated on an abstinent outpatient basis without the support of methadone or an antagonist did not do well. Before using antagonists we found our only successful treatments to be either residential treatment (e.g., Daytop) or methadone maintenance. We could not hold patients in outpatient abstinence therapy, as most became quickly readdicted.

Since clinical experience is not a substitute for controlled testing, we realize that to substantiate the above observations it will be necessary to compare three treatment programs: antagonist plus therapy, therapy alone, and antagonist alone. Only thus could we parcel out more adequately the relative contributions of each. We initially shied away from placebo studies for fear of overdose in unprotected individuals who would think they might be blockaded. We now feel that placebo studies would not provide an adequate test of the clinical efficacy of antagonists whose effects are only apparent when they are tested and which otherwise are not active agents. We therefore plan open studies with random assignment to the three conditions described above and patients knowing what they are on.

Although the retention rate has traditionally been one of the parameters considered in evaluating program success with narcotic addicts, it clearly is not one of the crucial outcome variables more closely related to success in the "real" world. Under this heading would be included employment or schooling, illegal drug use, other illegal activities as measured by arrest figures, and overall social adjustment. Most important, of course, is the behavior of these variables over time after individuals leave the program. We are still in the process of collecting follow-up data; until they can be reported, our main claims can only be that, with our antagonist programs as currently structured, individuals tend to remain in treatment, tend to do well while in treatment, and appear to have made good social adjustments after leaving us. We feel at present that these results are due to a combination of the therapeutic structure plus the antagonist, and that both are essential ingredients in the mixture. We further found that both antagonists have been tolerated well by patients, with few side effects—fewer with naloxone than with cyclazocine—and side effects that did occur essentially limited to the induction stage. Such findings suggest that antagonists can have a much wider use than they now have, both in the treatment of the adolescent addict not suitable for methadone maintenance and as an alternative to methadone for the older addict. Finally, our experience demonstrates that, once a program has experience with antagonists, outpatient induction is a very feasible proposition.

SUMMARY

The Drug Dependence Unit of the Connecticut Mental Health Center has been using narcotic antagonists clinically since February 1970. I have described two variants of a day program in which naloxone was used and an evening therapy group program in which cyclazocine was used. The day program gets around the shorter blockade (18 hours) of naloxone, while the evening program takes advantage of the 24- to 28-hour cyclazocine blockade. The holding power of the day program varied considerably with the therapeutic structure of the program, suggesting that, although the antagonist plays an important role, the therapeutic structure in which it is used is an essential variable. Both naloxone and cyclazocine were well tolerated by patients, had minimal side effects and these mostly limited to the induction period, and are viewed as useful adjuncts in the treatment of narcotic addicts. Although inpatient induction is recommended for programs just beginning with antagonists, once experience is gained outpatient induction is quite feasible.

REFERENCES

1. Chappell, J. N., Jaffe, J. H., & Senay, E. C. Cyclazocine in a multimodality treatment program: Comparative results. *Int. J. Addict.*, 6, 509–523, 1971.
2. Fink, M., Zaks, A., Sharoff, R. L., Mora, A., Bruner, A., Levit, S., & Freedman, A. M. Naloxone in heroin dependence. *Clin. Pharmacol. Ther.*, 9, 568–577, 1968.
3. Freedman, A. M., Fink, M., Sharoff, R., & Zaks, A. Clinical studies of cyclazocine in the treatment of narcotic addiction. *Amer. J. Psychiat.*, 124, 57–62, 1968.
4. Glasscote, R. M., Sussex, J. N., Jaffe, J. H., Ball, J. C., & Brill, L. *The treatment of drug abuse—Programs, problems, prospects*. Washington, D.C.: The Joint Information Service of the American Psychiatric Association, 1972.
5. Jasinski, D. R., Martin, W. R., & Sapira, J. D. Antagonism of the subjective, behavioral, pupillary and respiratory depressant effects of cyclazocine by naloxone. *Clin. Pharmacol. Ther.*, 9, 215–222, 1968.
6. Kleber, H. D. The New Haven methadone maintenance program. *Int. J. Addict.*, 5, 449–463, September, 1970.
7. Kleber, H. D., & Klerman, G. L. Current issues in methadone treatment of heroin dependence. *Medical Care*, 9, 379–382, 1971.
8. Meyer, R. E. *Guide to drug rehabilitation: A public health approach*. Boston: Beacon Press, 1972.

9. Pierson, P. S., Rapkin, R. M., & Kleber, H. D. Naloxone in the treatment of the heroin addicted adolescent. *Amer. J. Alcohol & Drug Abuse,* in press.
10. Wikler, A. Conditioning factors in opiate addiction and relapse. In D. M. Wilner & G. G. Kasselbaum (Eds.), *Narcotics.* New York: McGraw-Hill, 1965.
11. Wikler, A. Some implications of conditioning therapy for problems of drug abuse. *Behav. Sci.,* 16, 92–97, 1971.
12. Zaks, A., Jones, T., Fink, M., & Freedman, A. M. Naloxone treatment of opiate dependence, a progress report. *JAMA,* 215, 2108–2110, 1971.

PART III PRESIDENTIAL ADDRESS

INTRODUCTION

Joseph Zubin
New York Department of Mental Hygiene

I would like to point out first of all that Dr. Freedman's stance—that of the "middle range" outlook on narcotic addiction—is really out of character. I have rarely before seen him assume such a dispassionate stance. He is usually found at one extreme of an issue or the other passionately pursuing goals, usually for uplifting the fallen or freeing the underprivileged. This new, dispassionate, fence-sitting role ill becomes him, yet there seems to be a good justification for his position.

The middle-range outlook, like sitting on the fence, invites brickbats from all sides but also gives an unobstructed view of the scene below. What does our fence-sitter see? A striking panorama of "social, chemical, pharmacologic, psychologic, psychiatric, legal, and political forces" interacting with each other in a most intricate network so that it is almost impossible to separate primary from secondary factors, causes from effects. Some of these forces, however, seem to be better supplied and better reinforced than others. Thus, as far as governmental support is concerned, the chemical, pharmacologic, legal, and political forces have the upper hand while, until recently, the social-cultural forces were almost completely neglected. Yet, our biochemistry hasn't changed all that much in the past decade to explain the drug explosion and, if anything, our legal and political forces have served to increase rather than decrease the drug explosion. This puzzles Dr. Freedman greatly, and his paper demonstrates the appalling results of stressing only a few of the options that we could investigate to determine the causes of our drug era.

Our 20th century has comprised several eras, to which various moods have been attached. First was the era of anxiety, fanned by several world wars. Then began the era of depression in the post-sputnik period, and now we have an era of reveling in mood alteration reflected in the use of drugs. Social philosophers have tried to point out that during our anxiety era we really were not more prone to anxiety than our predecessors. The difficulty was that the institutions we established to assuage and contain anxiety had begun to fail. We lost faith in them and had not yet found substitutes. The drop in religious belief, the rise in divorce rate, the loosening of social structure—all influenced man's anxieties, and without new institutions to replace or bolster the tottering ones, anxiety increased.

We probably had no increase in *proneness to* depression either but, here again, the usual avenues for containing depressive moods and disorders apparently failed to assuage the hopelessness and futility of life faced by the atomic bomb.

How did the drug era develop? First it is important to distinguish between the so-called hard drugs, such as heroin and cocaine, and drugs such as marijuana and LSD which have different histories. Leaving aside the difficult issue of whether or not there has been a great increase in the number of individuals addicted to opiates, the characteristics of the addicted population have changed dramatically over the last 60 to 70 years. At the beginning of this century, the majority of addicted persons were white, middle-aged, middle-class southern women. Today the majority of addicts are black young males from deprived backgrounds. The use of marijuana, of psychedelics, of "ups" and "downs" by our population of youth is a new phenomenon altogether. The reasons for these trends are unclear, but they certainly do not lie in changed metabolism or chemistry of the human body in this period. For this reason, it is essential that studies of the ecological forces underlying drug use become a focus of our concern. The few studies conducted in this area have demonstrated, for example, that such factors as precocious maturity, peer-group and friendship patterns, rather than parental influence, are probably very influential in the spread of drug usage. Is it possible that our overcrowded schools, stress on watching rather than participating in sports, enforced schooling for a longer period—all conspire to turn our youth inward in search of self-stimulation for kicks? It is clear that such questions require a careful examination of the entire field from the vantage point that Dr. Freedman has taken.

NARCOTIC ADDICTION: THE MIDDLE-RANGE OUTLOOK

Alfred M. Freedman
New York Medical College

Not too long ago I was mugged in the doorway of my apartment building in New York City. I want to discuss briefly that experience because it has some small bearing on the outlook on narcotic addiction. One thing it does not do is give one the calm, leisurely, long or middle-range view.

As a matter of fact, being tossed to the ground, roughed up, and robbed—and all so fast that I never even saw my assailant—was a deflating experience. Fortunately, my ego was far more bruised than I was. And I had fantasies of revenge—if only I had carried a gun, or if I had an attack dog as so many people have these days.

But it was the assumptions made by others that shook me out of my Walter Mitty daydreams.

Everyone told me that my assailant was black and an addict. That was the conclusion of a policeman, a neighbor, a faculty member, and anyone else I told about the mugging. But since I did not see the mugger, I could not say. I felt a sense of irritation when any number of people said—quite sympathetically, I should add—"Ah, well, one of your addicts finally caught up with you!"

The area of narcotic addiction is of such complexity that all blind and unproved assumptions seem to me to present a danger in themselves that we, the scientific community of the American College of Neuropsychopharmacology, would do well to examine. Understanding requires opportunities such as this meeting, which allows our many viewpoints—in and out of academia and government—to delve into the many disciplines represented here: biochemistry, psychology, psychiatry, pharmacology, and neurophysiology, to name a few. There are also socioeconomic, cultural, anthropological factors to consider. And last, but hardly least, there are political considerations.

Narcotic addiction must be viewed in its context, in what I like to call the psychoecology [6, 7] of all drug use and abuse. Only in that way can we hope to achieve any true understanding (as scientists, researchers or practitioners, and as "addictionists"), hoping as we all do to devise successful prevention and treatment models and to help bring about the social rehabilitation of those human beings who are addicted.

In recent years I have devoted a good deal of time and energy to the development of heroin antagonists [8, 14]. These drugs will prove to be extremely useful, once they have been made sufficiently long-acting. My colleagues and I will continue to devote considerable attention to research developments of these drugs.

But I do not believe that the entire answer to heroin addiction is likely to come from cyclazocine, naloxone, or EN1639A administration. Any such notion is purest fantasy. Neither is the problem going to be solved by the morning methadone lineup.

And any momentary fantasy I might indulge that a single solution might in some marvelous way prove to be an answer to narcotic addiction is always brought up short by many illustrations: For example, the magic of penicillin has not eliminated syphilis.

I would prefer at this time to discuss the wider social implications of the drug abuse problem as an aspect of psychoecology—of which heroin addiction is the most disproportionate attention-grabber. The safer long view is not my topic today.

There is enough in the middle-range outlook that is both complex and perplexing, and there are problems that worry me considerably: issues, half-truths, even self-delusions that somehow victimize all of us.

THE NEW YORK CITY ADDICTS REGISTER

It is extremely difficult to obtain accurate statistics on the actual number of addicts in the United States. Figures are based on deaths from overdoses, arrests, and other approximations. Consequently, for some years I have looked to the New York City Addicts Register as a source of information [5]. The Register is not a perfect instrument but, all the same, it has been a serious effort to gain as accurate an idea as possible of the number of addicts in New York City.

The Register was begun in 1963. By 1967, approximately 35,000 addicts had been registered. In 1968, the total mounted to 58,000, and in 1969 this rose to 95,000. But, curiously, there has been no official report from the Register since 1969.

I have been told that there are "technical difficulties." At the same time, however, about 35,000 new addicts have been added to the Register each year. Of these, 25% or more are under the age of 20. A sixfold increase in the number of addicts has been suggested.

Knowing these figures, one can view some Department of Health statistics in a different light. According to the New York City Department of Health, only some 37% of narcotics-related deaths were among those on the rolls of the Register. And this, furthermore, suggests that the probable 200,000 or more names on the Register represent only about one-third to one-half of the heroin addicts in New York City. It is conceivable then that the actual number of heroin addicts may be approaching 600,000.

So the statistics may be telling quite a different story, just as we are boasting of the numbers enrolled in treatment programs and how the "epidemic" is tapering off or, at least, seems to have receded from its crest.

Without accurate data in these matters there cannot be an unclouded middle-range outlook on heroin addiction today. Even if the epidemic growth of heroin addiction has stopped, as some recent research suggests, there will still be a reservoir of opiate users. And our future plans about how to tackle the entire treatment problem or, more important, how to prevent the creation of more addicts, will depend on a realistic estimate of the numbers involved. At this point, we get contradictory signals or no data at all.

THE CRISIS OF CONFIDENCE

My dismay with the Register is part of a larger concern, the possible "discreditation" of the very disciplines that are represented in the American College of Neuropsychopharmacology. All scientists, including the medical specialists, are now faced with the consequences of instilling high hopes for the cure of disease. Many made ready promises believing they were necessary to convince a legislature or the Congress. But now we are reaping the whirlwind, and in many unexpected ways.

For instance, in 1966 and just recently, a Harris poll [10] ascertained what percentage of the public expressed "great confidence" in various professional groups. Percentages sagged sharply for scientists as a group, falling from 56 to 37%. For nonpsychiatric MDs, there was a drop from 72 to 48%; for psychiatrists the confidence decline was slightly steeper, from 51 to 31%. Not as many people had found psychiatrists as trustworthy as other doctors in 1966, and the comparison is still unfavorable to psychiatrists in 1972.

In fact, there has been a general decline of confidence in all leaders in all areas. Trust in members of the U.S. Supreme Court, once as high as for psychiatrists, has gone down even further, from 51 to 28%. I think we must be particularly concerned about the drop in the fields represented by our organization, and about the reasons for this state of affairs. We may have assured this loss of confidence by appearing to promise what we cannot possibly deliver. In the field of addiction there have been far too many vocal advocates of the one-and-only approaches. We have been focusing on one modality alone, when drug addiction is a very complex social, chemical, pharmacologic, psychologic, psychiatric, legal, political phenomenon. We have concentrated on narcotic addiction alone, and have largely failed to relate the hot issue of heroin to other drugs of abuse.

There has been not only a peculiar tunnel vision, but also an absolutely lethal interdisciplinary infighting. As a result, we have all become losers, and what we have done for the human beings who are addicted is examined—scornfully, may I add—by public and professionals alike. Only in this field could a meeting be called to examine treatment and legal practices under the title, "Discrimination and the Addict [3]." I am especially disturbed that we who profess to be healers are being regarded as if we were Mack the Knife. This dissonance cannot simply be explained by a conveniently aroused consumerism. We need to address ourselves to four basic questions we have so far largely failed to explore.

Question 1: Is Heroin Addiction a Social Problem Subject to Technical Solution?

I think not, is my first response to this question. Pharmacological substances that influence emotions are just too firmly imbedded in our lives. With a large reservoir of heroin addicts, it seems to me, the future will see repeated resurgences of addiction in cycles very much like the Asian flu. (See Musto, this volume.)

I do know that one can no longer even study a promising new experimental drug for the treatment of schizophrenia as if it were a neat, isolated clinical research project. That package deal has to be examined in all its aspects—moral, ethical, social, cultural, legal. And I know that there is no other area where these diverse factors are as compelling in their interconnection as in the psychoecology of heroin addiction. The lesson we learn here will serve us in understanding all subsequent problems we choose to tackle.

Still, that does not answer the question: Can a complex social problem find a happy solution at the hands of the modern technobureaucrats—those experts we know, love, and often depend on for our research grants?

We need them, they need us. But while bureaucrats are supposed to eliminate from all their official business any trace of love, hatred, the purely personal, the self-serving, the irrational, or any emotion, this has yet to happen. Neither has the bureaucratic machinery developed the utmost in speed, discretion, or the hoped-for reduction of personal friction. That is what Max Weber proposes; reality disposes otherwise, I suspect.

Technobureaucrats [9] play an increasingly important role in our society, even if often—too often—they can neither make the policy nor implement it, except with short-run solutions based on engineering models dealing with variables that are specifiable, interactions that are predictable, and modalities that can be quantified.

That a complex social problem has a potential technical solution is a bit of euphoria, I fear, that dates back to the halcyon Camelot days of John F. Kennedy. In a famous Yale commencement speech he claimed that we really know all we need to know, and that application of appropriate techniques would solve all existing problems.

But can the systems approach of a bureaucracy cope with the complexities of a human service system? That remains to be seen.

The technobureaucrats cannot make policy. In fact, a reluctance to make a policy or plan ahead is characteristic of political leadership in this country in general; thus, when we deal with a bureaucracy that is part of a political entity, rational planning becomes almost impossible. In fact, it is the seemingly inadvertent, frequently subliminal politicalization of the drug abuse treatment field that should be the cause of greatest concern.

Question 2: What are our Avowed as Opposed to our Real Goals?

Were I to attempt to ask all scientists, researchers or practitioners in the field, the so-called "addictionists," what they deem to be the number one priority, I dare say I would hear all about developing successful treatment models or methods and about social rehabilitation. Invariably, though, the foremost concern would be the individual therapeutic intention, with the main objective the betterment of the addict. There are those, of course, who will emphasize prevention and will not be satisfied until we have total prophylaxis, with no one ever abusing *any* sort of drug.

Yet while we formulate these priorities to each other, what is on the agenda of those who prompt or sponsor all our research and treatment efforts, of those in political power who formulate public policy? What does the public consider our number one priority?

Crime is on their minds. Any close scrutiny will bear this out. Irrespective of political party and with full-hearted support of public and press, the government at all levels worries mainly about crime and addiction as they proliferate together.

Certainly in recent years the great concern with crime connected to drug abuse has included the curious notion that all crime is committed by addicts [12]. This delusion is cherished by the public, politicians, and official agencies alike. The first effectiveness statistics hopefully offered by a new or even an old established drug abuse program invariably involve a pronouncement about a drop in crimes by its addict-patients. Very little is ever said about the quality of life led by those who have been successfully treated. This, of course, influences the researcher and therapist in the field of heroin addiction. He may believe that his work is therapeutic, but his expectations and often his pronouncements center on "good" crime statistics. He is thus the mystified victim of at least one unexamined assumption in the field of heroin addiction.

There is no doubt that addicts commit crimes; but how many is a matter of conjecture. Unknown is the extent of addict crimes solely to support the habit. We do know, however, that one-half to three-quarters of one group of addicts studied were delinquent before becoming addicted; in another study, 60% who tried heroin and 73% who became addicted had previous police records. It is simplistic, in any case, to presume that once heroin addiction was wiped out, crime would disappear.

We must not allow such expectations to make a sufficiently difficult task more complex. In the middle-range outlook on narcotic addiction, I regard this as one of the grave problems in the field. Therapeutic intervention will not, in fact, eliminate mugging and homicide from the streets of New York City. Crime remains and is related to many other factors.

It is important to remember that the Hudson Institute [13] estimated that no more than 500 million dollars a year is lost in New York City in all manners of thievery, by addicts and nonaddicts. This differs from the dramatic guesses that each year billions are ripped off by addicts alone.

Despite appearances to the contrary, we are not in the law and order business; but it is hard to tell, especially when a program cites a reduction of arrests as an achievement of treatment, as methadone or drug-free programs have done. On a methadone program's claim, the *New York Times* made an editorial comment [2], noting that the "relationship between arrests and crimes has to be considered simple and direct; thus, the study's revelation that addicts in methadone treatment commit far fewer crimes strongly implies that to expand methadone treatment programs is to make the city safer still." This again is an assumption presumed to be a fact.

We need increasingly to probe presumed facts, to ask ourselves the following questions:

Are we aware of our covert agenda as we should be? Are we aware of our *true* purposes in providing treatment to addict-patients? And, if not, are our avowed treatment programs doomed to failure? We need to learn the lesson of complexity, a bitter postgraduate seminar in a field of forces that many of us never suspected to exist.

Question 3: Can Aid or Comfort be Derived from Proposed Changes in the Narcotic Laws?

That is a moot point. Yet there is no real room for optimism here, either. Again the legal leaders of drug-law reforms take a very narrow view. So-called sensible reforms of our narcotics laws would deny probation in federal courts to any convicted heroin or cocaine trafficker while he is awaiting sentence or the outcome of an appeal. They would also place upon a defendant in federal narcotics cases the burden of convincing the court that his release on bail would pose no danger to another person. And they would provide for mandatory sentences for first-time drug traffickers.

HEW official Mervin Duval [1] has said that

there are some who will condemn reforms like this. They'll say it's taking a cops-and-robbers approach to drug-abuse control. But these critics haven't thought the problem through. Either that or they may be more interested in making political hay than in solving the drug epidemic. The tightening up and reform of our narcotics laws is not an attempt to take a pure enforcement approach to the drug problem.

It is an effort to solve the drug problem through proven public health techniques of case-finding, isolation, treatment, and cure. That's the way we have attacked the VD epidemic. Find out who has the disease, treat them, cure them. Every case treated and cured prevented a score of new cases . . . . That's not enforcement strategy. That's a public health strategy.

Experience has shown that enforcement offers us little hope of effective control, no matter what that approach is. And perhaps Dr. Duval is unaware that present approaches to VD, which he cites, have helped create a pandemic from a mere epidemic. We must assume that sensible reforms in our narcotics laws are not in the offing, despite the fact that legal approaches are repeatedly found unsuccessful, if not counterproductive.

Dealing with Drug Abuse. A Report to the Ford Foundation [15] stated:

> Public policy will never be completely successful in eliminating heroin use in the United States and the consequent street crime. Indeed, past reliance on law-enforcement measures has accompanied an epidemic growth of the heroin-addict population. It is ironic that our national policy, by resorting almost exclusively to criminal sanctions to eliminate addiction, has bred a thriving illegal market that can be sustained only by criminal activity.

The report cites two primary factors that impede public policy designed to suppress the supply of heroin: First, a very small amount of opium is needed to supply the U.S. demand for heroin (only about 2% of the total world production), which can be satisfied by the cultivation of just about 5 square miles of opium fields; and second, "The profits earned in domestic distribution are so great that it is unlikely the risks can be raised high enough to force dealers out of business."

Our field is subject to the unanticipated consequences of a single action, like methadone's unexpected seepage to the black market. In the area of enforcement, it seems to be the repeated seizing of heroin by the police that causes first a shortage, then an inevitable heroin price rise and, with it, increased addict crime. This might be called a counterproductive police action.

Question 4: What May We Expect from the Future?

Just now, legal approaches, administrative and social attitudes, and statutory laws all serve to obstruct the treatment of narcotic addicts throughout our nation. Also, we divert the public attention by the twirling of statistics, cops-and-robbers games of the French connection type, and competing prima donnas of treatment methodologies. What the middle-range outlook really needs is a comprehensive examination of the sociopolitical atmosphere in which all our efforts take place.

1. Innovation and enrichment of treatment methods. We need to develop a differential treatment program in which a number of modalities are available, each appropriate to the individual addict. The specific modality is to be tested in

the cauldron of critical evaluation of outcome. As psychopharmacologists, we should give high priority to the development of long-acting forms of a pure antagonist and long-acting forms of methadone. With the long-acting antagonists, one would aim for products that might be effective for weeks or months.

2. The development of methods of early intervention. We need to know a good deal more about the moment or act of beginning heroin use. Further, as the work in Chicago of Hughes and associates [11] has shown, the early period is the time of greatest involvement of others in addiction. It is the novice users who involve the uninitiated in addiction.

3. Since it is the very early period that is most infectious, the development of effective preventive methods is critical. We must head off the initial experimentation with heroin if we are to reduce and perhaps eliminate the steady recruitment of young people to the world of opiates.

4. We need fresh methods of involving the community, the most active participation in changing public attitudes, particularly of the young, toward heroin use, and their enthusiastic cooperation in coping with drug problems.

Perhaps we will get lucky—a great spontaneous cure will arise as a result of some outside event, for which we can, nonetheless, take all the credit. I have in mind the way in which the defeat of the crusaders and their expulsion from the Holy Land cut off the Middle East and so once and for all ended leprosy in Europe [4]. But it seems unlikely that such a miracle will happen. So it behooves us to pursue our treatment programs and short- and long-term research.

REFERENCES

1. Duval, M. K. Drug abuse control—more than money. Paper presented at the Annual Leadership Conference, American Health Association, New York, November 1972.
2. Editorial. *The New York Times*, Sept. 6, 1972.
3. First National Conference on Discrimination and the Addict, Washington, D.C., June 16–17, 1972.
4. Foucault, M. *Madness and civilization*. New York: Pantheon Books, 1965.
5. Freedman, A. M. The adolescent heroin drug abuse epidemic in New York City: 1949– ? Paper presented at the Fifth World Congress of Psychiatry, Mexico City, December 1971.
6. Freedman, A. M. Drugs and society: An ecological approach. *Journal of Comparative Psychiatry* , 13, 411–420, 1972.
7. Freedman, A. M. Youthful drug abuse. In L. Miller (Ed.), *Mental health in rapid social change*. Jerusalem: Academic Press, 1972.
8. Freedman, A. M., Fink, M., Sharoff, R., & Zaks, A. Cyclazocine and methadone in narcotic addiction. *JAMA*, 191, 202, 1967.
9. Gurvitch, G. *The social framework of knowledge*. New York: Harper & Row, 1971.
10. Harris Poll. *New York Post*, Nov. 13, 1972, p. 10.
11. Hughes, P. H., Senay, E. C., & Parker, R. The medical management of a heroin epidemic. *Archives of General Psychiatry*, 27, 585–593, 1972.
12. Markham, J. Heroin hunger may not a mugger make. *N.Y. Times Magazine*, Mar. 18, 1973, p. 38.

13. Policy analysis for New York state on drug abuse. Croton-on-Hudson, N.Y.: Hudson Institute, May 1970. (Mimeographed report)
14. Resnick, R. B., Fink, M., & Freedman, A. M. Cyclazocine treatment of opiate dependence: a progress report. *Comprehensive Psych.*, 12, 491, 1971.
15. Ward, P. M., & Hutt, P. B. *Dealing with drug abuse. A report to the Ford Foundation.* New York: Praeger, 1972.

OPIATE ADDICTION:
ORIGINS AND TREATMENT

AUTHOR INDEX

Numbers in brackets refer to reference citation in the text. Numbers in italics refer to the pages on which the complete references are cited.

A

Abbiss, S., 61 [29], *73*
Adler, F. L., 52, *55*, 176 [2], *183*
Adler, T. K., 27 [38], *42*, 53, *57*
Aigner, T. G., 63 [25], 66 [25], *73*
Alexander, K. R., 14 [53], *21*
Algeri, S., 103 [6], 106 [1, 10], *117, 118*
Axelrod, J., 15 [1], *19*, 26, 28, *40*
Azarasvili, A. A., 65 [11], *73*
Azmitia, E. C., 106, *117*
Azrin, N. H., 85, *90*
Azzi, R., 79 [2], *90*

B

Bagley, S. K., 61 [22], *73*
Bain, G., 32 [23], 33, *41*
Baker, B. R., 53 [2], *55*
Ball, J. C., 176 [2], 177 [3], 178 [3],
  180 [1], 182 [1], *183*, 211 [4], *219*
Balster, R. L., 62 [18], 64 [18], 65 [18],
  66 [16, 17, 18], 67 [18], 69 [18],
  70 [17], 71 [17], *73*, 79, 82 [5], 83
  [3], *90*
Barnett, R. J., 110 [15], *118*
Barry, H., 63 [2], 64 [1, 3, 4], 65 [1, 2,
  3, 4], 68 [26,], 69 [27], *72, 73*

Baumgarten, H. G., 108, *117*
Bednarezyk, H. J., 104 [50], *120*
Bell, E. C., 17 [7a], *19*, 65 [20], 68 [20],
  73
Belleville, R. E., 17 [2], *19*, 68 [5], *72*
Berger, B., 70 [6], *72*
Berzins, J. I., 17 [23], *20*
Bewley, T. H., 142 [2], 143, 144, *160*
Bhargava, H. N., 53 [3, 16], 54 [3], *55,
  56*, 106 [5, 16], 104 [16], 113 [4],
  117
Bishop, E. S., 95 [2], *97*
Blachly, P. H., 185, 186, *200, 201*
Blake, D. E., 106, *118*
Bliss, D. K., 63 [7], 65 [7], *72*
Bloom, F. E., 103 [6], *117*
Blumberg, H. H., 148, *160*
Borison, H. L., 13 [33], *20*
Bowden, C. L., 191, *201*
Bowers, M. B., 106 [7], *117*
Bowling, C. E., 17 [31], *20*
Boyle, W. E., Jr., 100 [49], *119*
Bradshaw, P. W., 61 [29], *73*
Bransby, E. R., 144, 146, 147, *160*
Brill, L., 177 [3], 178 [3], *183*, 204 [9],
  209, 211 [4], *219*
Brodie, B. B., 105, 110 [17], *118, 119,
  120*

SUBJECT INDEX

A

Abstinence, 8, 9, 12, 13, 15, 16, 29, 105
Acetylcholine, 14, 54, 102, 105, 116
d-Actinomycin, 52
Adenosine 3', 5'-cyclic monophosphate
  (cAMP), 109–116
Adenyl cyclase, 109, 110, 112, 113
"Affinity labeling," 53
Agonist, 13, 26, 49, 86, 204, 205
Alcohol, 15, 62, 64, 72, 94, 165, 182
Alpha-methylparatyrosine (AMPT), 84,
  105
Amines, 105
γ-Amino butyric acid (GABA), 115, 116
Amphetamines, 15, 47, 53, 69, 84–86,
  159, 182, 213
Antagonists, 16, 18, 26, 47, 50–52, 69,
  80, 84, 86, 131, 132, 166, 167,
  173, 203–208, 211–219, 226, 232
Antigen, 31, 32, 52
Antimuscarinics, 62, 66, 67
Antinicotinics, 67
Ataxia, 62
Atropine, 14

B

Barbiturates, 15, 68, 69, 79, 86, 94, 165,
  182, 213

l-BC 2605, 50
Benzodiazepines, 67
Blockade, 14, 17, 18, 52–54
Bucuculline, 116

C

Caffeine, 67
Cannabis, 15, 156
  (See also Marijuana)
Cataracts, lenticular, 29
Catecholamines, 14, 29, 53, 103–105,
  112
C^{14}, 38
  -dopamine, 38
  -tyrosine, 38, 104
P-Chlorophenylalanine, 29, 107–109,
  116
Cholinesterase inhibition, 102, 103,
  105
Cocaine, 15, 79, 86, 87, 94, 141, 142,
  156, 182, 213, 224, 230
Codeine, 27, 79, 80, 83, 86, 87
Conditioning, 8–19, 77–90, 129
  classical, 77–90, 129
  of drug effects, 13
  operant, 12, 77–90
Convulsants, 67
Cyclazocine, 50, 51, 84, 165, 173,
  203–208, 212, 216, 217, 219,
  226

N

Nalorphine, 9, 12, 15, 26, 27, 80, 84,
86–88
Naloxone, 50, 51, 100–116, 165, 204,
205, 207, 212–219, 226
Naltrexone, 207
Narcotic analgesics, 23–40, 59, 60
N-dealkylase, 26
N-demethylase, 26–28
New York City Addicts Register, 226, 227
NIMH, 43, 45, 50, 54
NIMH Addiction Research Center
Inventory, 205
Norepinephrine, 38, 54, 102–105, 112,
116
Normorphine, 26, 27

O

Office of Economic Opportunity, 166
Offspring of addicted mothers, 45, 55

P

Pain-pleasure principle, 7, 15
Pargyline, 105, 106, 112
Pennsylvania Department of Probation and
Parole, 176
Pentazocine, 86
Pethidine, 155
Philadelphia Teen Challenge, 176, 178
Phosphodiesterase, 109, 110
Physostigmine, 102, 105
Propiramfumarate, 86
d-Propoxyphene, 86
Propoxyphene, 79
Propranolol, 14
Psychedelic drugs, 18, 19

R

Racemorphan, 87
Receptor-induction theory, 28
Receptor-occupation hypothesis, 24

RNA, 54

S

Saline, 9, 83, 84, 87, 88, 102, 108, 112
Scopolamine, 67
Serotonin, 29, 54, 102, 103, 105, 106,
115, 116
Special Action Office for Drug Abuse
Prevention, 51, 124, 166
State-dependent learning, 17, 18, 59,
61–72

T

Theophylline, 111
Thymectomy, 52
neonatal, 35, 36
T-maze, 62–72
Tolbutamide, 14
Tolerance, 23–40, 43–55, 63, 79, 82,
85, 99–117
Treatment modalities, 128, 231
benign maintenance:
specific defect, 128, 129,
131–133, 166, 176–179,
203, 211, 212, 218, 230
character restructuring:
self-regulating therapeutic
community, 129, 131–133,
165, 176, 178, 203, 211, 218
conditioning antagonist, 129, 131,
203–208, 211–219
faith and dedication, 130, 131
medical distributive, 128
psychotherapeutic, 130–132, 176,
179
supervisory deterrent, 129, 131
Tryptophan, 108, 109, 115, 116

V

Veterans Administration, 50

W

World Health Organization, 7, 8